MORAL INJURY

MORAL INJURY

Mhairi Haarsager, M.D.

MORAL INJURY

Mhairi Haarsager, M.D.

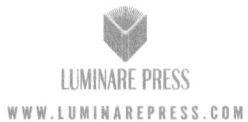

LUMINARE PRESS
WWW.LUMINAREPRESS.COM

Moral Injury
Copyright © 2023 by Mhairi Haarsager, M.D.

All rights reserved. This book or any portion thereof may not be reproduced or used in any manner whatsoever without the express written permission of the publisher, except for the use of brief quotations in a book review.

Printed in the United States of America

Luminare Press
442 Charnelton St.
Eugene, OR 97401
www.luminarepress.com

LCCN: 2023916494
ISBN: 979-8-88679-382-6

*Dedicated to the memory of Jane Graham Wild, WRNS.
1922–2014. Codebreaker, WW2. Trained at Bletchley Park.
Stationed in Colombo, Sri Lanka.*

Morally injurious experiences are defined as perpetrating, failing to prevent, or witnessing acts that transgress deeply held moral beliefs and expectations. Injury may lead to negative emotions and cognitions including guilt, shame, and lack of self-forgiveness.

Prologue

November 1954

She tiptoed around the small room, apparently absorbed in unnecessary tasks, keeping her father under close observation. Of the six people living in the house, she seemed always to be the first to sense when his dangerous rages were building. Of course, at nine years of age she was the eldest and most experienced, but her sister, only two years younger, was always absent when the terrifying rows erupted.

The pin began to slide from the grenade about fifteen minutes ago, when her mother, again, brought up the ancient electric stove with only two functioning plates. The suggestion that she calls in someone to fix it set him off. Pappa did not welcome visitors, particularly those who might diminish his authority by achieving something he had not.

Now her mother was upstairs bathing her brothers. Once they were settled in bed would Mamma venture back downstairs or go straight to bed? There were no locks on the flimsy doors and anyway, she'd seen him punch or kick holes in them before. So, the whereabouts of her mother would not alter the outcome, just the timing.

Until that time arrived, she must maintain her state of high vigilance in readiness to intervene. She was lonely, angry, afraid and, because she loved both Pappa and Mamma, she was sad.

In healthcare, moral injury may occur when healthcare professionals are asked to violate their judgment, in service to the financial needs of hospitals, insurers, or the government, rendering them unable to provide high-quality care. (Wendy Dean, Reframing Clinician Distress: Moral Injury, not Burnout. Fed. Pract. 2019 September; 36(9):400-402).

Chapter 1

Friday, December 19th, 1986

AT SHORTLY PAST TWO A.M. DR. LUSSI SIM WAS AWOKEN by an urgent call from Children's Hospital. This was particularly jolting because it was unexpected – she was not on call tonight.

The call was from Ann Castle, a senior transport nurse, who had flown by helicopter to a local referral hospital to stabilize a sick newborn for transport back to Children's Hospital. Ann was attempting to move the patient to the waiting helicopter but was being prevented from doing so by the referring physician, who did not agree with her patient care plan. After a short, blunt phone conversation with this physician, Lussi persuaded him that it was in his best interests to relinquish medical responsibility for the patient to her and allow Ann to proceed with the transport.

Endeavoring to disturb her husband as little as possible, she'd left the bed feeling lifeless and leaden; her brain striving for the clarity of function necessary to care for the desperately ill patient awaiting her. Before she left home Lussi called the neonatology fellow on night duty in the Children's Hospital Neonatal Intensive Care Unit, to discuss an interim patient care plan covering the period when she would be driving to the hospital and out of telephone contact.

Lussi's fondness for Baltimore had steadily grown over the decade she had lived here – however, after dusk, the streets of southeast Baltimore seemed to her to adopt a foreboding quality. In the anemic light from the street-lamps, the endless blocks of faux-stone row houses created a sallow, deserted stage set, camouflaging shadowy backstage alleyways.

As she slowed for a traffic light, Lussi reflected on the appalling fate of a mother driving her twin boys to daycare last week.

It happened at this intersection. She was murdered in front of her children in the crossfire between drug gangs. Violence is endemic in this city – a looming menace.

While balancing the brake and clutch with her feet and yearning for the traffic light to change, an uproar of screams and shouting invaded Lussi's head. Despite having suffered from these occurrences since childhood, her body tensed and she could feel sweat trickling between her breasts and shoulder blades as the threats, bellowed in foul, demeaning language, mounted in ferocity.

Lussi took her foot off the brake and accelerated through the red light. The din faded as she drove away from the intersection toward the Children's Hospital.

So far, she had encountered almost no other vehicles, but suddenly her driving mirror was entirely occupied by the front end of a large automobile.

Lussi abruptly accelerated, but the car behind took little time to catch-up.

Now there's a huge black limousine riding my bumper. The headlights are blinding. Pull yourself together, Lussi – why would a drug dealer be tailing you?

As Lussi turned into the hospital the black limo followed. The entrance to the employee parking garage loomed ahead. There'd been an armed abduction from this garage last month. Two teenage girls held the victim at gunpoint as she unlocked her car. The girls, later identified as outpatients on the adolescent medicine service, would have stolen this physician's vehicle if they'd been able to drive a car with a stick shift. Instead, one of them pressed a gun barrel into the nape of her neck and demanded that she drive to a "fucking ATM" and withdraw cash for them. The girls stole the victim's purse and made it clear they knew where she lived and that she had young children.

For some time after the abduction, Lussi's family had been inundated with concerned calls from friends and colleagues who feared it was she who was kidnapped. Like the actual victim, Lussi was in her mid-forties and one of the few members of the medical staff who drove a car without automatic transmission.

Lussi drove past the garage entrance and headed for the Emergency Room, which also housed the security office. The black limo was nowhere in sight as she got out of her car and glanced back at the garage. She ran into the security office to quickly report what she was able to discern of the limo's license plate number. Assured by the duty officer that he would immediately investigate the problem and that her car was not blocking ambulance access, she hurried to the Neonatal Intensive Care Unit.

On entering the NICU scrub room, Lussi found Ann Castle scrubbing her forearms and hands. It was clear from her smudged mascara and red-rimmed eyes that she'd been crying.

Drying her arms, Ann stepped off the faucet pedal and said, "I'm so sorry for dragging you out of bed when you are not on call, Lussi. You must have raced to get here so quickly. As I told you on the phone, this was originally a transfer for cardiology, but after I read the patient's birth history, examined him, and looked at his X-rays, it was clear he had meconium aspiration pneumonia. Following the instruction that Dr. Wright, the cardiologist on call, had given me – to give him prostaglandin, would only have made his condition worse.

"When I called Dr. Wright to explain why I didn't think the baby had a heart condition, I am pretty sure she hung up on me – I tried several times to reconnect, but only got a busy signal. Dr. Morrison is on call for the NICU tonight and is in the hospital. Normally I would have called her, but she's been stuck in the OR dealing with a baby with spina bifida who coded during a shunt procedure."

Grabbing a sterile brush to begin scrubbing, Lussi said, "Don't apologize for doing the right thing, Ann. I'm just sorry you got caught up in this mess."

"It was strange, Lussi, I've worked with her multiple times and Dr. Wright has always been respectful of my diagnostic abilities. But this time she was *so* certain the baby had a heart problem she didn't seem to want to listen."

"It seems odd that Sally Wright would make a major misdiagnosis like this. Had she been over to South Baltimore Hospital and examined the baby herself?"

"No. I didn't find out until I arrived at South Baltimore that she made the diagnosis over the phone."

"Oh. I see. Let's go look at the baby." Lussi said, putting on a gown and then using her elbows to open the door to the NICU. She and Ann headed to the ECMO Room.

On entering, the relative quiet of the NICU evaporated. The patient lay on his back on an infant warmer – motionless, except for the passive rise and fall of his chest with each strident ventilator breath. Intravenous lines ran into his umbilicus and left hand. Secured to both cheeks with tape, an endotracheal tube protruded from his mouth and was attached to the ventilator by a length of corrugated tubing. Multiple monitors, arranged in an arc behind the warmer, flashed, beeped, and sporadically alarmed. A pump technician was on her knees on the floor checking the connections on the ECMO – Extracorporeal Membrane Oxygenator pump system, prior to priming the circuit with oxygenated blood. The bedside nurse was slowly injecting medication into one of the IV lines and the fellow was intently watching a monitor tracing while she did so.

Looking back through the glass doors, Lussi could see that two surgeons were now in the scrub room, preparing to place the cannulas into the patient's neck vessels that would allow oxygenized blood to perfuse his bloodstream.

The fellow turned to Lussi as she reached the warmer bed.

"Hi, Dr. Sim. Thanks for getting here so quickly. Oliver here gave us a bit of a scare when he arrived – his oxygen saturation and his blood pressure fell during his transfer from the helicopter. We now have him restabilized on one hundred percent oxygen and high ventilator settings."

Lussi walked over to the X-ray viewing board on the wall and studied the images.

She turned to Ann. "Well, there is no question Oliver suffered some stress during delivery which caused him to pass, then aspirate, meconium stool into his lungs. His X-ray shows the classic findings of meconium aspiration pneumonia. Well done, Ann!"

"I obtained informed consent from Oliver's parents to put their son on ECMO, by phone." said the fellow. "They are dependent on a neighbor for transport. She's driving them here from South Baltimore, but she had to go home on the way to check on her own kids."

Lussi began her examination of baby Oliver Turner. Oliver was a full-term infant weighing seven pounds, six ounces. Despite his critical clinical status, he was a handsome baby, without remarkable birth-related bruising and with unusually lush curly red hair. Lussi had just finished listening to his chest when the surgeons entered the room and, with Ann's assistance, proceeded to don sterile gowns.

"Good morning gentlemen." Lussi smiled at the surgeons and moved back from the infant warmer. "I'll let you in here and conclude my examination when you've completed the cannulation. The faster we get the patient onto the ECMO pump, the sooner we can back off on his ventilator settings and reduce the barotrauma to his lungs."

Ann was about to leave for home and Lussi had just begun to review Oliver's medical records from South Baltimore Hospital, when Joe Meridian, M.D., Division Head of Pediatric Cardiology, appeared outside the ECMO room door dressed in street clothes.

Opening the door, a crack, Joe asked lightheartedly, "Been having some excitement out there in the trenches, eh, Ann? Good for the soul, I always say." Handsome, with a compelling personality, Joe was demonstrating his renowned and unshakable bonhomie, despite the hour. Lussi felt a familiar mix of emotions – envy of Joe's nocturnal vitality, and self-doubt. *Joe never seems to be tired or stressed. I wish I knew his secret. He's a great friend and colleague, but he shouldn't make light of Ann's traumatic experience at South Baltimore Hospital.*

She gestured to Ann and Joe. "Shall we meet outside to talk?"

Once outside the NICU, seated in a quiet corner, Lussi said, "Joe, Ann tells me she was informed by Sally Wright that this baby, Oliver Turner, had a heart defect and should be admitted to the cardiology service. Did the referring physician provide Sally with bad information?"

Joe shifted in his seat and stroked his chin. "Well, South Baltimore Hospital has just opened their NICU, Lussi, and I'm not sure how experienced their physicians are at referring patients to other hospitals. They started out working with their own cardiologists but, apparently, neither of them was trained in this country and they couldn't provide documentation that their training met United States medical licensing requirements. I received a call from our esteemed CEO, Bill Schultz, a couple of weeks ago, asking if our service would step into the void and take consultation calls from the South Baltimore NICU until they can hire permanent cardiologists. This is their first emergency transfer, and it seems they waited far too long to call us. Sally Wright couldn't drive over there fast enough to examine the infant before the transport team arrived."

"I've just been hearing from Ann about the outrageous way she was treated at South Baltimore, Joe. The doctor there was aggressive, unprofessional, and, most importantly, he was wrong. We owe it to Ann that we have a live patient. I intend to file a complaint with their Chief Medical Officer and hope that you will back me up."

Staring at the floor, Joe said, "I can only apologize profusely to both you and Ann on behalf of Sally. To be fair to her, she told me the referring doctor sounded knowledgeable about the patient and emphasized to her that there was a strong family history of male infants with hypoplastic left heart defects. She said the way that he presented the case over the phone made it sound as though the baby had a heart problem. However, she admits she did not question him adequately about the birth history, partly because the infant sounded so sick and obviously needed urgent intervention. She's very embarrassed by her error, so I came in to see what I can do to set things straight."

"It doesn't sound like you've heard the whole story, Joe. I am sure that Ann will be happy to fill you in on the reasons that 'fairness to Sally Wright' is hardly a priority item on our agenda." Lussi nodded in Ann's direction.

"I have *never* experienced anything like this before, Joe, and believe me, I've learned to deal with arrogance and sexism on the job. The doctor at South Baltimore was *absolutely determined* to make me give prostaglandin. He was so aggressive I thought he was going to attack me." Ann paused.

"So, I called Dr. Wright at home, explained the diagnostic problem, and expected her to speak to the doctor and back me up. But, instead of that, without explaining her reasoning, she insisted I obey him and give the prostaglandin. Then she hung up on me. I was astounded. She knows me well – I have transported patients for cardiology for almost eight years.

"So, then I called the fellow on-call for our NICU. He agreed with me that I shouldn't give the prostaglandin and should get the patient over to Children's as soon as possible. Unfortunately, as soon as the respiratory therapist and I got ready to move the patient out to the helicopter, the referring doctor called a security guard to prevent us from leaving. That is when I called Dr. Sim because Dr. Morrison could not leave the OR."

"You are correct, Lussi – I did not have the full picture." For a rare moment, Joe seemed lost for words. Then his face relaxed as he said, "Ann, the behavior you were subjected to during this transport *was* unacceptable and, I promise you, I will follow through with those involved. However, as it turns out, it's a good thing the patient is now on the neonatology service because it seems he's a definite candidate for ECMO. I would like to get together as soon as possible with you both, to discuss how that excellent outreach teaching program of yours can help us improve the medical skills of the NICU staff at South Baltimore."

Lussi grimaced as she responded to Joe's last point. "It's not just their medical skills that need improving, Joe. They urgently need an in-depth course on how to communicate in a professional manner.

"On top of that, their patient charting is terrible. For example, there is almost no documentation of the labor and delivery, the baby's status at birth, or his condition during the period in their NICU before Ann and the respiratory therapist placed him on the ventilator. As a result, I won't be able to give Oliver's parents a fully informed assessment of whether he might have suffered injury from his low blood oxygen levels. This cannot be allowed to happen again, Joe."

It was after eight a.m. by the time that Lussi had reviewed the results of Oliver Turner's laboratory tests, ultrasounds, and X-rays, supervised his placement on ECMO, and talked to his parents. In twenty minutes, she had to start patient rounds with the NICU team, and before that, she should move her car into the parking garage.

"Hi Doc," called an officer as Lussi passed the open door of the security office, "I haven't been able to track down the vehicle that was following you. I checked the plate information you gave me, and it doesn't fit with any of the faculty license plates we have listed. I also searched the staff parking garage without any luck. Are you sure it was a Maryland license plate?"

Lussi smiled, "Yes officer, I'm certain. Thank you so much for checking, but please don't spend any more time on it. I've been a little nervous since the abduction from the garage and I overreacted to being followed so closely."

I really must get hold of myself – lighten up and control my imagination.

Chapter 2

Friday, December 19th, 1986, 7:55 a.m.

WHEN BILL SCHULTZ, CEO OF CHILDREN'S HOSPITAL, arrived at work with Suzanne Sinclair, his CFO and regular commuting companion, he was frowning ominously. He parked the car, then punched the steering wheel several times before getting out. Suzanne had noted his brooding, distracted manner when he picked her up at her home, a contemporary suburban mansion conveniently located next door to his own substantial property in Howard County, Maryland.

When Bill was in an expansive mood, Suzanne could count on a drive to work that began with what Bill described as "stratospheric" sex, consummated on the soft leather rear seats of his S500 Mercedes. That this liaison took place less than a mile from their unsuspecting spouses, he'd informed her, added significant titillation. She was aware that her relationship with Bill had become an ongoing source of hospital gossip, but had gained the impression that his wife, Donna, had lost interest in keeping tabs on him.

Today there was no erotic interlude to lighten their commute. Bill completed the drive in brooding silence.

As they walked together from the parking garage to the hospital entrance, Bill finally exploded, "Fuck. These goddamned people seem to think I was appointed as their nursemaid. Did you see that editorial in yesterday's *Sun*?

According to the loser who wrote it, 'several' members of the medical staff stated that the recent staff abduction would not have happened if I had agreed to have panic buttons installed in the garage. I ask you, who gets held up by *teenage girls*, and why the hell can't the adolescent medicine people control their patients?"

As they entered the hospital atrium, Suzanne risked a tentative response. "The girls did have a loaded gun and substantial criminal records, Bill." Bill snorted and marched into an elevator.

Not that it would matter to Bill – and she carefully avoided any tell-tale body language, but Suzanne particularly loathed this side of his personality. She characterized such outbursts as infantile tantrums, resulting from his pampered upbringing as the only son of the *Chargé d'affairs* for the United States Embassy in Riyadh, Saudi Arabia. He went to school with Saudi princes and readily bonded with their affluent lifestyles.

Bill had been CEO of Children's Hospital since nineteen eighty-four; two and a half years. But both their affair and their working relationship began earlier when he was CEO of a large community hospital in Texas. His predecessor at Children's was an internationally respected professor of pediatric infectious diseases, who adhered to the key principle propounded by the hospital founders – that the hospital should provide excellent care to all children, regardless of the ability of their family to pay for it. The board of directors at Children's had ousted this professor without warning, in favor of a CEO who fully embraced the prevalent fiscal concept that all hospitals should be run as for-profit corporations.

Suzanne was aware, from experience, that her attempt to cool Bill's anger against the medical staff had served only to redirect it onto herself. In his eyes, she had failed to show him the respect he believed he deserved by omitting to enthusiastically agree with his derogatory remarks.

After all, to him, I was just a low-level financial officer at the hospital in Texas when he 'persuaded' me to move to Baltimore with the promise of promotion to CFO. Tolerating his numerous defects is just part of the job.

As Suzanne entered the fifth-floor office suite, Bill was loudly berating his office manager. She had, apparently, allowed Tony Blake, the hospital COO, to wait in Bill's office without an appointment. Before Suzanne reached the door to her office, Bill turned to her abruptly. "Ms. Sinclair, you will join us *now*, in my office."

Suzanne had a meeting scheduled for eight fifteen but sharing this fact with Bill was a waste of time. She unlocked her office door and threw her coat on a chair. On the way to Bill's office at the other end of the suite, she asked the office manager to cancel this appointment and reschedule.

As one of Bill's hand-picked henchmen, Tony Blake, M.D. enjoyed multiple fringe benefits in addition to his generous salary and bonuses. From Suzanne's observations, these included free rein to tyrannize the hospital staff. Although not demonstrating the empathy or dedication to the care of children desirable in a pediatrician, Tony had been the Director of Pediatric Intensive Care prior to his promotion. Arrogant and aggressively ambitious, his personality seemed to precisely fill Bill's requirements for a COO, but Tony was highly unpopular with the more than eighty percent of faculty members whom Bill characterized as "whining sheep."

Although Suzanne was close behind Bill as he entered his office, he did not hold the door open for her. Immediately he was across the threshold he gruffly commanded, "Tell me what it is you wish me to do for you, Tony."

Bill's thick gold bracelet clinked against his Rolex as he reached up to hang his jacket on a hook behind the door. Rolling up his shirt sleeves, he crossed the spacious office to his oversized desk; past walls plastered with photographs of himself greeting celebrities and dignitaries.

Tony, who was pacing the room, had slung his suit jacket on the back of one of the two chairs in front of Bill's desk. Suzanne took the other chair, with no acknowledgment from Bill.

Standing, with his hands on the back of his chair, Tony finally responded, "Well Bill, there was a fuckup last night with the first cardiology admission from South Baltimore Community Hospital. One of our cardiologists diagnosed congenital heart disease, but the transport nurse deduced that the patient didn't have heart disease. This nurse called Lussi Sim and reported that she was being pressured by the South Baltimore doctor to administer a drug that could seriously harm the patient. The result is that the patient was admitted to the neonatology service rather than cardiology, and I have that bitch, Lussi Sim, in my face about quality of patient care and systems failure." Tony sat down heavily next to Suzanne.

"Jesus!" Bill sprang out of his chair and loomed over his desk at Tony. "Where the hell *was* this cardiologist? Their contract with South Baltimore states that they *must* go in person to the referring hospital to consult on patients prior to transfer. I doubt the transport nurse would have dared to argue face-to-face with an attending cardiologist."

"Sally Wright is the cardiologist in question, Bill. She told me that the patient's condition was rapidly deteriorating, and he needed helicopter transport. She couldn't get to Children's from home in time to ride with the transport team on the helicopter, nor could she drive to South Baltimore Hospital fast enough to examine the patient before the team got there. So, she made the diagnosis over the phone."

Tony instinctively ducked as Bill grabbed a marble obelisk from his desktop, cradling it contemplatively in both hands. "Tony, I made it quite clear to you that the cardiologists were to admit these patients to their service without question *even if they disagreed*, when a heart condition was diagnosed by a referring physician at South Baltimore. Also, I would remind you, all our medical staff are required to live within ten miles of the hospital."

Tony interjected. "I made those requisites quite clear to Joe Meridian, both before and after the event, Bill. He did initially demur on the requirement not to question the diagnosis but agreed that the patient could then be reassessed on admission to Children's. I guess we both overlooked the fact that the transport nurse oversees the administering of drugs required to stabilize the patient for transport. Of course, if Dr. Wright had gone to see the patient as she was supposed to, she could have postponed giving the prostaglandin until the patient was admitted to Children's. However, this was the first patient transfer from a brand-new hospital. I'm certain that Joe will make sure that things go better in the future. Maybe this could be considered a trial run, Bill?"

Suzanne could not avoid visibly flinching as the obelisk left Bill's grasp and crashed into the front of an antique display cabinet on the opposite side of the room. "Trial run? We're not talking about training the high school football team here, Tony. We get things right from the get-go. Why do I pay you the big bucks, Tony? To make sure that things go as I want them to, right? Right? Get out of my office and don't return until you have dealt with this problem."

The office manager, in search of the source of the loud crash, almost collided with Tony as he hurried from the office. Suzanne admired her calm demeanor, as she retrieved the obelisk and examined the display cabinet.

She'd do well in my line of work.

As Suzanne left, before closing the office door behind her, she heard Bill bark at his manager, "Get hold of Joe Meridian. Tell him I want to see him immediately, in my office. Then get me on the line to that moron Don Evans at South Baltimore and bring me some coffee."

Chapter 3

Friday, December 19th, 1986, 8:20 a.m.

HURRIEDLY ENTERING THE SCRUB ROOM FOR THE SECOND time that day, Lussi came to a sudden halt.

This place is filthy!

Despite constant exhortation by the hospital's most senior infection control nurse, who had become an almost permanent fixture in the NICU over the past few months, the scrub room was clearly underserviced. The sinks and floor were soiled, there were puddles of water on the floor, the waste receptacle was overflowing and, because the routine, morning restocking of the cupboard above the scrub sink hadn't been done, Lussi had to use the intercom to request a scrub brush from the desk clerk and ask her to put in an urgent call for cleaning staff.

As she scrubbed, Lussi reviewed the six months since Bill Schultz held what he termed, a "Town Meeting," to present the state of the hospital's finances. At this meeting, Schultz had warned that there would be "major cutbacks," but had not specified what these cutbacks would be. Not surprising to anyone who had experienced them before, the initial cutbacks primarily targeted the nursing and janitorial staff, resulting in a significant reduction in numbers, expansion of individual job descriptions, and a substantial decline in morale.

It had not done anything to bolster Lussi's optimism that, at the same time the number of essential hospital staff was shrinking, the executive hospital management, in abrogation of the hospital mission but with the blessing of the board of directors, was pushing forward with the development of upscale specialty outpatient clinics. These clinics were specifically located in areas around the beltway where the inhabitants were upper middle class or above, and sufficiently far from the hospital that patients in the hospital service area would have limited access due to transport issues.

Approximately two months after the town meeting, a headline appeared in the city section of the *Baltimore Sun: Despite Job Cuts Hospital Executives Vote Themselves Bonuses*. According to the article, senior administrators at Children's Hospital would receive a total of three hundred and seventy-five thousand dollars in bonuses. Tony Blake had taken pains to emphasize to the reporter that these bonuses were less than the amounts received in previous years. Tony rejected any suggestion that, in view of the hospital's financial situation and the recent announcement that the workforce was to be cut by a further ten percent, he and the other senior executives might consider forgoing the bonus payments. He stated that these executives needed the bonus because they were demoralized by the shrinking workforce and reduced hospital services.

The rounds that Lussi was about to lead in the NICU this morning would be multidisciplinary. Held twice a week, on Mondays and Fridays, the usual daily team on rounds; attending physician, intern, pediatric resident, fellow (neonatologist in training), and neonatal nurse practitioner, were joined by a nutritionist, a pharmacist, and a nurse educator. Rounding involved a detailed review of each patient at their bedside and usually lasted over two hours.

For review today was the customary cohort of extremely small premature infants with multiple medical problems. These tiny humans were almost invisible beneath the mass of lines and tubes connecting them to noisy therapeutic and monitoring devices. There was also an assortment of larger and more mature infants, including some that were on the cardiology and surgical services. During rounds, the patient's primary nurse and the pediatric resident or nurse practitioner caring for them would provide an update. The group rounding would then discuss and adjust the treatment plan going forward.

With every patient Lussi paid great attention to detail, reviewing overnight records, and gently examining each baby herself. She loved bedside teaching, and the feedback she received indicated that this was appreciated by her team.

As she rounded, Lussi was always gratified to see how meticulously the babies were cared for by their primary nurses. The smallest 'preemies', weighing from seven hundred and fifty grams to fifteen hundred grams, were optimally positioned and supported, each one wearing a miniature pair of handmade sunglasses to protect their eyes from the NICU lighting, which was never turned off. Their multiple tubes and intravenous lines were individually labeled. Infant warmers and incubators were clean and free of debris from therapeutic procedures. These nurses vigilantly guarded their fragile patients against any potentially harmful intrusion.

The rounds ended in the ECMO room. Although residents and nurse practitioners were not involved in the care of the infants on ECMO, they would inherit these patients once they were weaned from the pump.

Presenting Oliver Turner, the fellow told the team, "Oliver's clinical status is critical but stable. During labor, Oliver responded to unknown stress by passing meconium stool in utero and inhaling a large amount of meconium-contaminated amniotic fluid, causing meconium aspiration pneumonia. This led to increased back pressure in the arteries in his lungs which, in turn, prevented adequate circulation of blood through his lungs and a severe drop in his blood oxygen levels. The ECMO pump is a miniature cardiac bypass machine. It supplies oxygen to Oliver's organs that his lungs cannot provide. As his condition improves, the technician will gradually decrease the flow of oxygenated blood to him from the pump."

"What is the baby's prognosis?" the resident asked.

"Since Oliver's admission, we have received sparse clinical information from the referring hospital," Lussi explained. "We know he is the first live birth; his mother has had two miscarriages. But she was scheduled to have a normal spontaneous vaginal delivery this time, which suggests that an uneventful pregnancy was anticipated. However, when her waters broke, there was meconium in the amniotic fluid and the fetal heart monitoring tracing showed signs of fetal distress, which can cause a fetus to gasp and pass stool. Because of these findings, Oliver was delivered by emergency cesarean section.

"At birth, the obstetrician gave him reasonably good Apgar scores of six out of ten at one minute, eight out of ten at five minutes, and nine out of ten at ten minutes of life. These acceptable scores were, however, contradicted by a note in the nursing record describing Oliver's condition at birth as 'pale and floppy', and stating that he did not start breathing spontaneously until six minutes after birth. This description certainly does not match with his assigned Apgar scores which, even if his heart rate was normal at birth and his color improved with oxygen, could not have been higher than two at one minute and four at five minutes of life.

"So, in answer to your question, Oliver's prognosis is uncertain at this juncture and, unfortunately, this is all I could tell his parents. He has responded well to ECMO so far, so I currently have no reason to be overly pessimistic."

Chapter 4

Friday, December 19th, 1986, 7:00 p.m.

ON WEEKDAYS, THE SIM FAMILY SELDOM SAT DOWN TO dinner in their dining room. After-school commitments and unpredictable work hours meant staggered arrivals; easier to accommodate in the kitchen. Tonight, however, inclement weather discouraged even the most intrepid chionophile from leaving the house, allowing the opportunity to catch up with each other over an unhurried dinner.

Lussi heard a hunk of snow from the roof land with a thump outside.

Much as I love snow, I'm glad I'm not on call this weekend.

The conversation turned to plans for a ski trip to Norway at the end of January. Mumbling into her napkin, Lussi's thirteen-year-old daughter Rachel was almost inaudible. "Mom, is there any chance we could stay with Uncle Jens this time?" Rachel's brother, fifteen-year-old John, nodded in support.

Lussi took a bite of salmon absent-mindedly and swallowed it too fast. After a bout of coughing, she said, "Well Rachel, Uncle Jens has said many times that we're welcome to stay with them, but your grandmother will be so disappointed."

"But Uncle Jens lives close enough to Grandma and Grandpa that we can visit them every day. I just think that John and I annoy Grandpa, even though we try not to. Then he gets mad with Grandma and yells at her, and you get so stressed out, Mom."

"You guys don't annoy my father. He loves you both, but…"

Lussi's husband Howard interrupted. "Lussi, I think that Rachel is trying to say that she and John would like you to have a stress-free vacation. We've got plenty of time to discuss this over the weekend. For example, we could split the stay between your parents and Jens. Let's table this discussion for tonight and relax."

Howard, an ex-Navy seal, was six years Lussi's senior, in his early fifties. Tall and athletic, she admired how he kept himself in shape, especially since he got most of his exercise doing outdoor activities with his family, rather than in a gym. Howard was a medical research maven, based at the National Institutes of Health in Bethesda, Maryland. Trained in infectious diseases, his spectrum of special interest ranged from the development of new vaccines and therapeutic agents to internationally recognized expertise in agents of biological warfare.

Their daughter Rachel was close to a clone of Lussi. She was tall, freckled, and had long strawberry-blonde hair like her mother's. Rachel was intelligent, thoughtful, and studious, and Lussi considered her daughter far more creative and adventurous than herself. Rachel's brother, John, had a vibrant personality to match his bright red hair and an infectious sense of humor. Only an inch shorter than his father, he was smart, considerate, and inquisitive.

Lussi was relieved that their parents' demanding jobs didn't seem to adversely impact either child. She was forced to acknowledge, however, that work stress was affecting her own ability to relax and enjoy the other aspects of her life. *God. I have almost finished my second glass of wine but I continue to ruminate on the research paper I have to complete this week and the most critical patients in the NICU.*

"So, is everybody ready for *juleaften*?" Lussi enquired. "As a self-interested reminder, there are only four days to go before we open our presents on Christmas Eve, and I, for one, am very much looking forward to all the treasures that will be heaped upon me by you amazing guys."

Laughing, John said, "Over-the-top compliments will always work for me, Mom, and yes indeed, for once I have no need to grab my skis and bravely set off into the blizzard to search for goods and chattels fitting to present at the feet of my most cherished Mamma."

Howard, on the other hand, appeared somewhat sheepish. His face had taken on a hangdog expression. He slapped his forehead with the palm of his hand and said, "I knew I had forgotten something."

"Oh Dad, you say that every year," Rachel giggled. "We all know by now that this is a major falsehood. You are so organized you probably bought all your presents months ago."

"Well, I do have to admit that I slipped off my pedestal just a bit this year, Rachel. I didn't complete my shopping until the first week of December."

By now everyone was laughing.

As she finished her main course, Lussi silently chastised herself for feeling weighed down by work right now.

I signed up for better or for worse when I chose to specialize in intensive care. Doing my best for my patients has to come first and, despite the tension intrinsic to caring for sick babies and their families, I love working with the NICU staff to provide first-rate, compassionate care. I must admit, however, that winding myself up, almost daily, to argue with administrators who seem to care far more about the bottom line than the well-being of the patients, is taking a toll. Is it my body language? Somehow, I trigger their hostility before I even open my mouth. I wish I were better at hiding my feelings and could present a calm, amiable demeanor.

"Earth to Mom, Earth to Mom – come in!" John's voice broke into her thoughts. "You were really lost in the clouds, Mom. There is a rumor going around that there is apple pie and ice cream for dessert?"

"Oops – sorry! Yes indeed, this rumor is bona fide."

Later, when Rachel and John had left the table, Howard asked, "How are you doing dear?" Did the emergency last night have a happy ending? You seem a little remote this evening."

"I was scared driving into the hospital last night, Howard. I feel so stupid. Someone was tailgating me in a black limousine for the last few miles and I got thinking about that poor woman who was killed last week. The limo followed me onto the hospital campus before it disappeared—I thought into the parking garage, but the security guard couldn't find it there. I think I made a fool of myself with Security."

Howard's forehead creased with concern as he leaned toward her. "I don't see why you should think being afraid was stupid, Lussi, especially after all that has happened in the past few weeks. I worry about you every time you get called in at night. I hope the security people took the incident seriously."

"Security definitely took it seriously, Howard; I just wish the drive was the worst of it."

Lussi strove to organize her thoughts. "The on-call cardiologist made the wrong diagnosis on the baby we admitted last night. Luckily, Ann Castle was the transport nurse on duty. When Ann examined the infant at the referring hospital, she realized the diagnosis she'd been given by the cardiologist wasn't correct and refused to administer an inappropriate medication, even though the doctor there tried to intimidate her into giving it."

Howard's right arm shot toward Lussi's shoulder, spilling white wine onto the front of his sweater. "After all the effort that you and Ann have put into teaching the staff at area hospitals how to stabilize sick babies for transport, I didn't think this kind of thing could still happen. I'm so sorry, Lussi. *And* I'm a klutz."

Handing him a napkin, Lussi said, "This is a new hospital. Do you remember that hospital out near Columbia that was the center of a lot of controversy two years ago? The one they demolished so much low-income housing to build?"

"I do remember reading something in the newspaper and wondering why we needed another community hospital in the area."

"Well, they've opened a mid-level Neonatal Intensive Care Unit and our cardiologists are apparently doing consultations for them. It amazes me that they were given permission; I have a hefty non-compete clause in my contract with Children's Hospital.

"Anyway, according to Joe Meridian, who came in to cover for his colleague because, he said, she was too embarrassed to face us, this was the hospital's first referral of a baby to another hospital since their NICU opened. I don't feel that this is an acceptable excuse for their abysmally inadequate records of patient care from birth to hospital transfer. I had to talk to the parents without a detailed birth history, and the Apgar scores assigned didn't align with the description of the baby. I've tried to contact the obstetrician who delivered him, but he hasn't returned my calls."

"Wasn't the cardiology division at Children's in some sort of trouble around about the same time people were protesting the building of this hospital?"

"Yes; but that was the cardiac *surgery* division – specifically, the heart transplant program. The program failed an accreditation inspection; their surgical numbers and survival rates were low, and the rate of complications was high, so the regulators put them on probation. Since then, they've failed a re-inspection, so the regulators made Children's shut down the program."

"Sounds like a good thing they won't be doing any more transplants, Lussi."

Howard yawned and removed his damp sweater. "Let's forget work and have another glass of wine in front of the fire. We have a whole weekend off. The kids are putting the dishes in the dishwasher, and I refuse to even think about snow removal until tomorrow. I also hereby decree that you'll no longer dwell upon any of the events you've just described. I would've had the same response you did if someone had tailgated me in the middle of the night in that part of town. Involving security was totally appropriate in the circumstances. There's nothing you could have done to prevent the mix-up with the baby. You've told me that Joe Meridian is a great guy on multiple occasions; so many that I've wondered if I should be jealous. On this occasion, however, it seems he did not adequately prepare his team for a new consulting responsibility."

Lucy laughed. "There's no reason at all for jealousy Howard. Joe is a kind, supportive colleague who has gone out of his way to offer me assistance on occasions when I have really needed it. He is a good friend, that's all. Besides, he's married to a gorgeous blond.

"To tell you the truth, Howard, my mental state on that drive didn't help. I was stressed to begin with, so much so that I had one of my flashbacks before the black limo even entered the picture. I had thought that they were decreasing, but I've been having them more frequently in the past couple of months. And now the kids have opened-up about not wanting to stay with my parents. The walking-on-eggs atmosphere in their house, even now that my father is physically confined to a wheelchair, is unpleasant for them. I am so conflicted – guilty for exposing our children even to a watered-down version of what I experienced as a child, but also for robbing my poor mother of time spent with her grandchildren."

As they left the table, Howard put his arm around Lussi's waist and steered her in the direction of the couch.

"I am certain the kids are more concerned about how visits to your parents affect *you,* Lussi. They have more resilience than you credit them with, and they don't have the memories that weigh on you. We will work on a plan for Norway together. Now let's relax and enjoy the fact that we don't have to work tomorrow."

"You are right Howard. I don't know you put up with me being so tedious." Lussi sank back into the couch cushions with a sigh, "This is the life."

As he handed her a refilled glass of wine, Howard whispered in Lussi's ear. "May I also suggest that an early bed might further delight your senses, my love?"

Chapter 5

Monday, December 22nd, 1986, 7:30 a.m.

Lussi made it a habit to arrive at work early after a weekend off duty. She was in her office triaging phone messages. The second voicemail was from Ann Castle, requesting that Lussi meet with her before rounds began in the NICU, and asking if she was aware that the hospital had recently contracted with a company to supply agency nurses to work in the NICU. Lussi immediately called Ann. She also left a voice mail message for the NICU Director of Nursing, Muriel Dressing. Then, overcome by frustration, she sank back into her chair and stared at the ceiling.

Ann arrived three minutes later. Before she sat down, she asked, "Lussi, did senior management consult you about hiring these agency nurses?"

Lussi shook her head. "No, Ann, I haven't heard any mention of this. Have they completely lost their sanity upstairs?"

Ann rolled her eyes. "I thought not. It's appalling that they would do something like this without clearing it with the Medical Director of the NICU. As I said in my voicemail, I'm very concerned about the skill level of these nurses. They don't appear to be trained to safely perform even the most routine tasks in the NICU. Muriel met with senior NICU nurses last week to discuss the *remote* possibility, as she put it, that we might need to hire an occasional agency nurse if the census in the NICU remains so high. All of us thought it was a terrible idea and Muriel seemed to agree with us. When I arrived at work today, there was a memo in my inbox from Sherry Dunstan, our 'beloved' Chief of Nursing Services. In it, she informed me that I've been put in charge of the 'agency nurses assigned to work in the NICU.' This being the case, I am responsible for making sure that they have 'mastered all the required skills.'

"On top of this, it turns out that the contract with the agency officially started last Monday. Someone had already scheduled an agency nurse for the night shift on Saturday. I checked with the charge nurse who was on duty that night, and it turns out this agency nurse didn't even know how to check capillary blood sugar. Our nurses had to keep a constant eye on her – and this didn't go down well with the troops, particularly since one of their colleagues was reassigned to work the shift on a general pediatric ward just to accommodate this nurse. Muriel told me that it is guaranteed in the contract with the agency that their nurses will be assigned to work in the NICU."

"Has Muriel made her feelings clear to Sherry?" Lussi asked, expecting the worst.

"Yes, but apparently it went down like a lead balloon. She got both the, 'It's your job to correct any deficiencies' spiel and the 'management has determined that these nurses are competent, and everyone needs a little guidance at first in an unfamiliar unit' guff. A *little guidance?* Capillary blood glucose testing is a basic skill that all general pediatric RNs should possess, let alone the NICU nurses."

"I've asked Muriel to meet with me after rounds, Ann. Knowing her I'm pretty sure but, before I take this matter to the executive floor, I need to be certain she had no role in enabling management to employ these nurses without my knowledge. I've got to start rounds in the NICU now, but I promise I will get back to you on this before the end of the day."

As she entered the intensive care unit on her way to check the ECMO patients before NICU rounds began, Lussi was, as always, struck by the comfortable temperature and relative quiet. She'd completed her fellowship training in neonatology in the nineteen seventies when the ambient temperature in the NICU was kept high to compensate for the single-walled infant incubators. These incubators were significantly less efficient at retaining heat than modern, double-walled models. For the same reason, earlier NICUs housed all the patients in one room, so that those entering were assaulted by the heat and a cacophony of beeps, hissing, and strident alarms.

This modern NICU provided single and double patient rooms, based on the severity of the illness. The ECMO room was significantly larger than the others, to accommodate two patients, two primary nurses, two pump technicians, and two ECMO pumps.

When Lussi left the hospital on Friday evening there were two patients on ECMO, and there had been no ECMO admissions over the weekend. Oliver Turner was doing so well on Friday that Lussi wasn't surprised to find only one patient in the ECMO room. After reviewing and examining this patient, and writing orders, she asked his primary nurse if she knew the number of the room to which Oliver Turner had been transferred.

"You mean you haven't heard what happened, Dr. Sim? Oliver was doing well and was ready to be taken off the pump, but during morning rounds on Sunday his condition suddenly went downhill, and he died on Sunday afternoon."

"I'm sorry – what? How on Earth did this happen?"

"It was on my Sunday morning shift. The cardiology team consulted on Oliver and then moved on to examine this baby. Suddenly, Oliver's oxygen saturation dropped into the low eighties, and his blood pressure fell. Since the cardiology team was still in the room, they were able to start resuscitating him immediately. Dr. Sula also got back in here fast. He'd already examined both patients and left Oliver's bedside to round in the NICU just a short time before his condition worsened. Oliver seemed to respond a little after about twenty minutes of CPR, but the improvement didn't last."

"Thank you for the information. This is so unexpected." Lussi put a hand on the wall to steady herself – "I'm sorry – just a little dizzy." *His poor parents. I told them before I left on Friday that Oliver was doing well and should wean off ECMO quickly.*

"Are you OK, Dr. Sim?"

"Oh yes – yes, thanks I'm fine. This is a bit of a shock. It is unusual for an infant on ECMO to die so suddenly after showing steady improvement, but it could have been a bleeding complication caused by the anticoagulant medication he was receiving. Did the doctors say what they thought was causing Oliver's deterioration?"

"Dr. Sula said that the cardiologists thought Oliver had an open *ductus arteriosus*."

Lussi wished she could talk at once to her colleague, Dr. Azad Sula. However, in less than five minutes she had to start rounds with the NICU team – talking to Azad would have to wait.

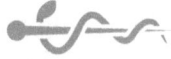

11:00 a.m.

THE OFFICE OF THE NURSING DIRECTOR OF THE NICU was located behind the central patient monitoring desk. Muriel Dressing was an attractive brunette in her late forties and, despite her petite stature, had a commanding presence. The staff in the NICU admired and respected her.

As Lussi knocked and entered her office, Muriel was on the phone, holding the receiver to her right ear, while supporting her drooping head with her left forearm as if she had a severe headache. "Yes, I realize that management expects us to explain the financial situation and the need to hire agency staff, but my nurses are asking questions I can't answer."

Muriel lifted her head, grimaced at the receiver, and indicated that Lussi should sit down. A few seconds later she hung up the phone with a sigh of exasperation. "Talk about heads in the sand, Lussi. No one upstairs seems to either want to know what's going on down here in the real world or help us to deal with it."

"Muriel, did you know in advance that the fifth floor was planning to contract with this nursing agency?" Lussi asked, endeavoring to remain calm.

"Yes, they alerted me about a week ago that they might have to hire some agency nurses because of the high census, but I was assured by Sherry Dunstan that the nurses in question were trained to work in the NICU. I've since heard from Ann Castle that her experience to date does not indicate that these nurses are adequately trained and that you didn't know anything about this plan. Even knowing what Sherry is capable of in terms of making bad decisions and ignoring our input, it never occurred to me that she would do something like this behind your back. I apologize sincerely for not asking if she'd talked to you. I felt sure she must have got your OK and I thought if you agreed to it, maybe her plan had redeeming features she didn't share with me."

Lussi was puzzled. "But what did you think was going to happen, Muriel, when our nurses found out that they might be replaced by agency nurses and rotated out of the NICU to work on the general wards?"

"When this plan was initially brought to my attention, it was all about having *additional* nursing staff to *assist* our nurses. However, since it turned out this was not an ad hoc contract for short-term coverage, I shared those very concerns with Sherry. She told me straight that my nurses would just have to deal with it, because of the hospital's financial problems. No room for negotiation."

"Do you mind if I talk to Sherry?"

"No Lussi. I would really appreciate your doing that." Muriel smiled for the first time.

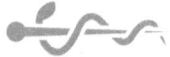

1.15 p.m.

As usual, as she made her way to the Executive Management Suite on the fifth floor, Lussi could feel her jaw tightening, her heart thumping, and her body tensing. She'd involuntarily fisted her hands, as she'd done from early childhood when forcing herself into a battle zone she really wanted to escape.

In her early days as a junior attending physician, Lussi had been happily unaware of the progressively for-profit approach to hospital management under adoption by the senior executives. When she joined the faculty at Children's, in the late nineteen seventies, the CEO had also been the Medical Director, an altruistic specialist in pediatric infectious diseases, who believed that all children deserved excellent medical care regardless of the socio-economic status of their family. Five years after Lussi joined the medical staff, this CEO/Medical Director was ousted by the board without ceremony, in favor of an MBA, sporting gold jewelry and a permanent suntan.

New appointments to the hospital board were now disproportionately allotted to local bankers and other corporate 'pillars of the community'. The current board did not value altruism; *Free care doesn't pay bills* was a favored discussion-quashing mantra used on the fifth floor.

That executive nurse management would always appropriately support the nursing staff was another misconception Lussi had held. Sherry Dunstan, Director of Nursing, was a nurse in name only. She'd stepped onto the management ladder immediately after completing her training as a registered nurse and rarely ventured onto a clinical unit. Staff hypothesized that she was afraid to get too close to the patients in case an emergency forced her to reveal her lack of practical nursing skills.

Via the active hospital rumor mill, Lussi was quite aware that Sherry regarded her as a nemesis; one of the members of the medical staff willing to go the extra mile for the nurses and to whom the nursing staff looked to present their perspective. It was also common knowledge among the nursing staff that Sherry viewed them as a feudal landlord would regard the peasants working on his estate. They were a necessary nuisance.

Lussi greeted Sherry with a smile she didn't feel. She'd learned since Bill Schultz became CEO, that Sherry had his strong backing and followed his directions without question. Feeling nauseatingly sycophantic, Lussi said, "Thank you Sherry for taking time out of your busy schedule to allow discussion of a significant problem." It was all she could do to stop herself from mentioning the underhanded process that precipitated the problem.

Sherry, a bony, spectacled woman of indeterminate age, with cropped iron-grey hair, tapped a pen on her desk throughout Lussi's review of the potential dangers to NICU patients posed by inadequately trained nurses. Lussi also voiced her support for Muriel Dressing and the NICU nursing staff, emphasizing that this was a risk management problem requiring urgent action.

Sherry leaned back, adjusting her glasses ponderously. "Well, Dr. Sim, you of all people should know that the general pediatric nurses regard the NICU nurses as whiners. They think they are superior to the general pediatric RNs and expect special treatment because they work in intensive care. I think it will do them good to supervise and teach these new nurses – bring their egos down to earth."

As if about to throw it, Sherry grasped her pen like an arrow. She then proceeded to repeatedly thrust it back and forth in Lussi's direction as she continued, "In view of the hospital's financial situation, the nursing staff should be happy they still have their jobs and benefits. I can assure you that Mr. Schultz is in full agreement with my views. He and I are not here to rearrange the deck chairs on the Titanic, we're here to stabilize the hospital finances so that we may continue to provide excellent patient care."

Once Sherry began to quote familiar mantras used by those on the fifth floor to suppress reasoned opposition, Lussi recognized that it was futile to argue or to point out that the potential malpractice suits resulting from the current situation were unlikely to enhance either the reputation or the financial stability of the hospital. Sherry would report to Bill Shultz as a threat, directed at the board of trustees and the hospital, *any* reference she made to the legal system. Bill had, with the blessing of the chairman of the board, abolished the formal lines of communication between the board members and the hospital staff, so she had no means of defending herself.

It was mid-afternoon before Lussi was able to leave the NICU to go to the Neonatology office suite. As the Division Director, Lussi supervised four other neonatologists, including Azad Sula. Stopping at her office manager's cubicle to check for recent messages, Lussi asked her if Dr. Sula currently had anyone in his office. Barbara Melnick had been her office manager for eighteen months, running things with easy-going expertise. She'd done wonders for office efficiency and made Neonatology the envy of other divisions.

Azad was at his desk signing patient discharge summaries when Lussi knocked and poked her head around his office door. He beckoned her in. "I can guess what you want to talk about, Lussi. The death of baby Turner took us all by surprise."

Lussi nodded. "What happened, Azad? What do you think caused him to deteriorate?"

"Well, that's a good question, Lussi. I examined him before NICU rounds started, and all seemed fine. I'd just left the ECMO room when I was paged to return. The cardiology team was already there, examining the other ECMO baby, when baby Turner's oxygen saturation fell to eighty percent and his heart rate dropped to forty beats per minute. By the time I arrived at his bedside, the cardiologists had begun resuscitation. They told me the baby's blood pressure had also dropped precipitously, and he had developed a heart murmur compatible with an open *ductus arteriosus*. An ultrasound confirmed the open ductus, and his chest X-ray was reported by radiology as showing either blood or excess fluid in his lungs."

"Was blood suctioned from his airway?"

"No. So we ruled out hemorrhage and worked on closing his ductus. He just didn't respond as I'd hoped. We tried to resuscitate him for almost an hour."

"I feel terrible, Azad," Lussi confessed. "On Friday, I told Oliver's parents that his prognosis was guardedly good."

"I can understand, Lussi. The parents were called in while we were attempting to resuscitate him, but they didn't arrive until after he was pronounced dead. They were in shock and did ask for you, but I explained that you were off duty for the weekend. I talked to them for some time, with the chaplain present."

"When is his autopsy being performed?"

"There won't be an autopsy. The mother couldn't bear the thought of it."

"But an autopsy is mandatory, Azad; this was an unexpected death that occurred within seventy-two hours of admission. Didn't you call the Medical Examiner?"

Before Azad could answer, Lussi's pager went off; an urgent call to the NICU. "I'll catch up with you later, Azad. We need to talk more about this." Lussi ran from the room.

"Room three!" A nurse shouted as Lussi entered the NICU.

The fellow and the senior pediatric resident were attempting to resuscitate an infant with skin the color of mottled grey marble; a nurse was suctioning white material from the baby's airway.

Over his shoulder, the fellow said, "One of the agency nurses placed a feeding tube but neglected to confirm that the tip was in the stomach before she put the formula into it. Turned out the tube was displaced into the airway, so she'd poured almost two ounces of formula into the baby's lungs before she noticed a problem. We've been working on the patient for about six minutes and, as you can see Lussi, we are still suctioning loads of formula out of her airway. We just gave intracardiac epinephrine for a heart rate under ten – it's up to thirty-two now."

For the next thirty-five minutes, Lussi worked with the team to save the patient; without success.

Chapter 6

Tuesday, December 23rd, 1986, 1:00 p.m

LUSSI WAS ON HER WAY TO MEET WITH DR. HUNTER, Chief Medical Officer, and Judy Stevens, Risk Manager, to review the case of the infant with the misplaced feeding tube. On entering the room, she was surprised to find Tony Blake, Dianna Stuart (in-house General Counsel), and Sherry Dustan seated in a row on the far side of the conference table. Already sweating and experiencing tightening in her chest, Lussi took a seat opposite them. Judy, Dr. Hunter, and Joe Meridian were helping themselves to the coffee set out on a sideboard.

A smiling Joe handed Lussi a cup of coffee and sat down next to her whispering, "Thought you might need a friend in court so, as a member of the risk management committee, I invited myself." Lussi felt her breathing ease a little as she thanked Joe for the coffee.

Dr. Hunter called the meeting to order and asked Judy Stevens to take minutes. Turning to Lussi, he said, "Dr. Sim, I realize that you expected to meet with just Judy and I, but Tony called me this afternoon about the problems with the baby transferred from South Baltimore Community Hospital and, since we already had this meeting set up to discuss another risk management problem in the NICU, I suggested he attend."

Tony Blake raised his hand and added, "Since both

problems involve nursing and risk management, I took the liberty of also inviting Sherry and Dianna."

Dr. Hunter asked Lussi to describe the problems surrounding the admission of Oliver Turner, referring to him as 'Baby T'.

Following Lussi's report on what transpired during the transfer of Baby T and the medical implications, Tony Blake was the first to comment. "Well, I'd say that we are in the clear when it comes to any legal issues, wouldn't you agree Dianna?"

Dianna carefully reorganized a small pile of documents in front of her, taking her time to reply. "Well Tony, I would strongly advise you to remember that this meeting was called to discuss quality improvement issues, rather than legal issues. If the meeting minutes do not make this clear, they will be legally discoverable should a suit be filed.

"Even though the transport team from Children's acquitted themselves appropriately, there's still the question of the initial failure to make the correct diagnosis. As Lussi just told us, had the transport nurse administered the prostaglandin prescribed by Dr. Wright, there's a real possibility that Baby T would have died as a result. In other words, this was a pretty close call."

"Yes, Dianna, but all of this is just teething problems with a new setup. These things take time to work out. Isn't that right, Joe?" Tony said, tipping back his chair and almost winking at Joe. "I'm sure there are lots of valid reasons why this type of thing could happen during the first patient transfer from a new hospital. Joe has assured me that he will make sure that, in the future, all his cardiologists will make every feasible attempt to personally examine the patient *prior* to transfer from South Baltimore Hospital."

"Correct Tony," Joe said. "Also, I intend to personally educate the pertinent staff at South Baltimore regarding the importance of making their referral calls as soon as possible so that our guys can get there, preferably with the transport team."

"Thanks, Joe. One more thing while on the topic of education. It seems to me that Dr. Sim has at her fingertips the cure for any lack of expertise on the part of the NICU staff at South Baltimore Hospital."

Tony turned to Lussi with a smirk on his face. "That expensive outreach education program that you use to train our competition, Dr. Sim; well, here's a great use for it. Get your team over there to South Baltimore and show them how to do things properly, eh? I'll call Don Evans, the CEO out there, and smooth your way."

He's going to do nothing about this – just dump the whole mess onto my lap.

Judy Stevens averted an irate response from Lussi by interjecting, "I'm sure that Dr. Sim is intending to do exactly what you are suggesting Tony, however," pausing briefly for emphasis, "I will complete my investigation into this matter and report back to Dr. Hunter as per protocol."

Tony's eyes flashed with anger that belied his calm response. "Yes, of course, Judy. Totally appropriate."

Lussi swallowed her temptation to remind Tony once again that the "expensive" outreach teaching program to which he was alluding was provided at no cost to the hospital. It was paid for by outside grant funding.

It's not worth it. I just must stay calm.

Joe took a leisurely sip of coffee and, staring directly into Tony's eyes, said, "I totally agree with Dr. Sim that this was a sloppy infant transfer. In retrospect, I should have taken the first call myself, but to tell you the truth I failed to recognize the urgent need for educational input at South Baltimore. I take full responsibility for the errors made and, if she is willing, I think it's a great idea to have Dr. Sim set up a program for the NICU staff at South Baltimore Hospital as soon as possible."

Ignoring Tony Blake's intimidating stare, Lussi smiled at Joe and said, "I can certainly do that Joe, but we need to include the Obstetric staff. Ann Castle and I will visit South Baltimore and draw up a priority curriculum, in cooperation with the staff there."

Dr. Hunter requested additional comments. None being proffered, he moved the discussion to the feeding tube incident. "Dr. Sim, please describe for us the incidents that you believe led to the death of this infant. For the purposes of the meeting minutes, Judy, we'll refer to this patient as 'Baby M.'"

"Thank you, Dr. Hunter. Baby M was a full-term infant admitted to our NICU yesterday, at the age of twenty-two hours. She was born with a congenital cyst under her tongue, known as a *Ranula*. The cyst didn't interfere with her breathing or swallowing but was large enough to prevent Baby M from completely closing her lips to suck. Because of this, she needed a feeding tube temporarily, until surgery could deal with the cyst. Baby M was entirely normal otherwise and had an excellent prognosis."

"How did an agency nurse come to be assigned to care for this infant, Lussi?" Judy asked.

"That's a key question, Judy. Baby M was full-term and the least sick patient in the NICU. Rather than having a new nurse with unknown skill level care for a critically ill infant, it was thought that an essentially well baby like Baby M would be a good initial patient for her.

"As not uncommonly happens with an active infant, Baby M's feeding tube was accidentally displaced during her transfer to our NICU. It was assumed, based upon information supplied by Sherry, that the agency nurses could safely perform routine healthcare procedures on infants."

Sherry Dustan's face reddened as Lussi continued, "The cyst in the baby's mouth did not increase the difficulty of replacing the tube, the agency nurse simply had no idea what she was doing and, as a result, failed to utilize a standard method to ensure the safe placement and use of a feeding tube, i.e., testing tube aspirate for stomach acid. Because she did not do this, she did not realize that the tip of the feeding tube was not in the stomach – it was in the patient's airway. She fed formula through the feeding tube into the patient's lungs. This was the direct cause of death.

"I should add that the decision to hire agency nurses for the NICU was made by senior administrators as a cost-cutting measure, without consulting me."

Sherry Dunstan abruptly left her seat and, adjusting her posture for maximum height and folding her arms, stared down at Lussi. "Well, I certainly hope that Dr. Sim is the only person in this room who is not aware that we must all pull together to address the hospital's financial problems. We care for a high percentage of non-insured patients. We must do the best we can with what we have."

Lussi could no longer contain her outrage. She stood, placed her hands on the tabletop, and leaned toward Sherry "Ms. Dunstan, if we are not able to provide optimal patient care the NICU should close. I can't believe that you're condoning this lethal and totally avoidable error based on hospital finances."

Dr. Hunter held up his hand and indicated that everyone should take their seats. Attempting to defuse the situation, he stated, "Clearly Dr. Sim is upset on behalf of this patient, and that is totally understandable. However, I'm sure that she'll agree that running a hospital is a complex undertaking and there was no evil intent underlying the hiring of what were, I understand, held out by the agency to be NICU competent nurses."

"'*First, do no harm.*' This imperative was drilled into me at medical school and I'm sure into you also, Dr. Hunter." Lussi could feel her face flushing. "I can't comment on evil intent, but I can state that, in my opinion, hiring nursing staff with unproven skill levels and promising them that they can work in one of the hospital units requiring the highest level of nursing skill is tantamount to gross medical negligence."

Tony resembled a rabid animal poised to leap across the table. As Dianna Stuart grabbed his shoulder and pulled him back into his seat, he pointed his index finger at Lussi and jabbed at the air. "Dr. Sim. We have all heard more than enough of your opinions. Because of your opinions, we no longer have a heart transplant program. All your sniveling about patients developing seizures, infections and God knows what else. Well let me tell you, the hospital board is not at all happy about losing the heart transplant program, and rest assured Dr. Sim, they've been kept updated on your unsolicited opinions."

Dr. Hunter hastily adjourned the meeting.

As he escorted Lussi from the room, Joe turned to her with a lopsided grin, and whispered, "Well, that probably could have gone better."

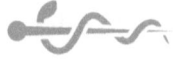

1.50 p.m.

Yesterday, Lussi had attempted to contact Oliver Turner's parents to express her condolences, but no one answered the phone. Once she returned to her office and took time to recover her equanimity, she tried again and got Mr. Turner on the line.

"Hello Mr. Turner, this is Dr. Sim, the doctor that spoke with you and your wife on Friday. I'm calling to let you know how very sorry I am that we were not able to save your son, Oliver."

"Yes, Dr. Sim, I remember that you were very kind, and my wife and I appreciate everything that was done for Oliver at Children's Hospital."

"I also wanted to ask if we can help you and your wife with funeral arrangements or in any other way. Have you received a call from our social work department?"

There was a prolonged pause, then Mr. Turner said, "It is so kind of you to call us, doctor. My wife is sleeping now, but she will be so comforted to hear that you called. We could tell when you talked to us that you really cared about Oliver, and we know that everyone did their best for him.

"We have decided not to have a funeral for Oliver because your colleague Dr. Sula told us that a funeral is very expensive, but the hospital will not charge us anything to cremate Oliver's body. Our Church is holding a memorial service for Oliver this weekend and I gave your social worker the place and time for anyone who would like to come."

"I very much appreciate the invitation, Mr. Turner, and I would like to attend."

"My wife will appreciate that. She wanted to thank you herself, but she is very sad just now. We did not get to the hospital before Oliver died and she was not allowed to hold him."

"Why – why couldn't she hold Oliver?"

"Dr. Sula told us that Oliver was on medicine that would make his blood leak out from the tubes in his body if he was taken off the ECMO machine."

What? That's crazy. Azad can't have said that. The cannulas are clamped to prevent bleeding and we always allow the parents to hold their baby in circumstances when nothing further can be done to save them.

"Would you like me to give you the date, time, and directions to our church, doctor?"

"That is very kind of you Mr. Turner, but I can get the information from Social Work. You and your wife need to concentrate on looking after each other."

Azad's refusal to disconnect Oliver's body from the ECMO pump and the ridiculous reason he gave Oliver's parents is bizarre. If the Turner family spoke a first language other than English or if Azad didn't have a perfect command of English, I might have considered the possibility that, due to the stress they were under, Oliver's parents might have misheard him – but neither of these factors pertains. It's been a terrible day and, after that catastrophic meeting yesterday, I'm not even sure I still have a job, but as soon as possible I must speak to Azad again.

Chapter 7

Wednesday, December 24th, 1986, 11:24 a.m.

LUSSI WAS IN THE HOSPITAL'S MAIN AUDITORIUM LISTENing to one of her second-year fellows conclude a case presentation at the monthly interdisciplinary Ethics Case Review.

She had not yet had the opportunity to follow up with Azad Sula. Barbara had informed her yesterday that he was out of the office for family reasons. Now he was seated several rows behind her. As soon as the conference concluded, Lussi positioned herself between Azad and the conference room door, so she could easily steer him aside.

Intercepting Azad as he attempted to edge himself around her into the crowd leaving the room, Lussi steered him to a relatively quiet spot close to the doorway. "Azad, I just need to clarify something with you. It will only take a minute." She began, as he again tried to maneuver his way to the exit.

"I called the Turner parents yesterday to see how they were coping." Despite her disbelief, Lussi held her ground as Azad put a hand on her shoulder and attempted to push her out of his way.

"I know it will sound ridiculous, Azad, but Oliver's parents think that you told them that his body couldn't be removed from the ECMO circuit because his blood would drain from his cannulas? His mother is extremely upset that she wasn't allowed to hold him. This doesn't make sense, and I'm pretty sure this can't be what you told them; or is it?"

Azad took a step backward. "No, Lussi, I certainly didn't say that. I did, however, tell the parents that, if they agreed to an autopsy, we would need to leave all the cannulas, tubes, and lines in their baby for the pathologist – which is standard procedure. Mrs. Turner was already very upset because Oliver's body was so swollen with fluid, and when I told her this, she refused the autopsy. She probably didn't clearly hear anything I said after that."

"But Mr. Turner heard the same thing, Azad. Can you explain that?"

"No, Lussi, I can't, but we both know that parents frequently mishear bad news."

"But it's our job to ensure that they understand, Azad. We also both know how much parents of dead or dying patients value being able to cuddle their baby, and there is absolutely no reason I can fathom that Oliver's body couldn't have been detached from the pump like we usually do. On top of that, why were you asking the parents for autopsy permission in the first place, when the case would have to be referred to the Coroner's Office?"

"I did call the Coroner's Office, Lussi, but they declined the case on the grounds that the baby was so ill on admission to the NICU that no additional data were required to explain his death."

At that point, Azad finally managed to finesse his way around Lussi and through the doorway. As he hurried away, he called over his shoulder, "Lussi, I'm sorry, I'm late for a meeting. Can we discuss this another time?"

"You bet we will," Lussi muttered under her breath.

On the way to her office, Lussi met Barbara waving a memo slip.

"I was going to stick this message on your door, Lussi. Dr. Blake called to say you will be welcomed at South Baltimore Community Hospital. The contact person will be the Director of Neonatology, Dr. Naeem Daher. His telephone number is on the message."

Well, I guess this might indicate that I'm not about to be fired.

Lussi read the message and handed it back. "Thanks, Barbara. Please would you see if you can get hold of Dr. Daher for me now? I'll be in my office."

Barbara nodded and smiled.

After she'd spoken to Dr. Daher and made an appointment to visit his NICU with Ann Castle after the Christmas vacation, Lussi called the Baltimore Medical Examiner's office. It did not take long to track down the pathologist who was on call the day that Oliver Turner died.

After introducing herself, Lussi asked, "I wonder if you remember receiving a call last weekend from Dr. Azad Sula at Children's Hospital, concerning an infant who had died while on ECMO?"

"Well, yes, I remember the call clearly. We receive relatively few calls regarding ECMO patients."

"Dr. Sula tells me that you declined the case; what was the reason?"

"As you know, as a Medical Examiner I must decide whether a death occurred under suspicious circumstances. That did not appear to be the case with this patient. He would have to be in a critical clinical status to be placed on ECMO in the first place so, logically, he was at high risk of dying. Although our protocol does state that our office should be called if a hospital patient dies within seventy-two hours of hospital admission, unless the death is totally unexpected, we usually do not choose to open a Coroner's case. This is especially so with infants – your hospital pathologists have much more experience with this age group than we do."

"Did you inform Dr. Sula that an autopsy by a Children's hospital pathologist was required?"

"Not in this case. As you know, even if we do decide that the circumstances of a patient death warrant opening a Coroner's inquiry, we will frequently ask your pediatric pathologists to perform the autopsy for us and send us the report. In this case, however, I remember that I told Dr. Azad to go ahead and ask the parents for autopsy permission because this was not an unexpected death. Are you calling because you think there were suspicious circumstances?"

"No, not at all. But this infant was doing so well on ECMO that his death came as a bit of a shock – I was just making sure that I had all the details for our mortality review. Thank you so much for your time, you have been extremely helpful."

Well, I guess that's that. No need to chase after Azad anymore. Why is he being so evasive?

Chapter 8

Tuesday, December 30th, 1986, 10:30 a.m.

Lussi was driving with Ann Castle to meet the NICU medical and nursing staff at South Baltimore Hospital for the first time.

From the outside, the hospital was a standard, mid-sized community hospital ostentatiously adorned with a massive, bronze *Caduceus* above the main entrance. Lussi considered the *Caduceus* an inappropriate symbol for a medical facility because, in mythology, the *Caduceus*, a winged staff with two snakes intertwined around it, is the symbol of the Greek god of thieves, merchants, and messengers, and of his Roman equivalent, Mercury, who is patron of thieves and outlaws.

The correct medical symbol is the *Rod of Asclepius*, the Greek god of medicine and healing. A wingless staff with a single snake wound around it.

Lussi was puzzled when, as a young physician, she arrived for the first time in the United States from Norway and encountered the *Caduceus* decorating hospitals, clinics, ambulances, and healthcare products. She'd initially ascribed the error to naïve confusion of similar symbols, but her subsequent experience with the American healthcare system had, occasionally, caused her to question whether the only naivety involved was her own.

Lussi and Ann entered an expansive marble lobby that resembled the shopping area of a luxury cruise liner, boasting, among other amenities, classy gift shops and an upscale hairdressing establishment. A tall, bearded man with dark hair greying at the temples hurried over from a bank of elevators to greet them. He was wearing green scrubs under his white coat, and expensive sneakers.

Dr. Naeem Daher shook hands enthusiastically with both Lussi and Ann, but simply nodded in the direction of a pretty, blond woman standing behind him, as he introduced her as the Nurse Director of the NICU without providing her name. The Nurse Director acknowledged his introduction with a shy smile but did not move or speak.

After they'd toured the Labor and Delivery suite and the NICU, Ann left with the Nurse Director to meet with the NICU nursing staff. Lussi and Dr. Daher adjourned to his surprisingly cramped office, so filled with textbooks and piles of medical journals there was little space left for his desk and two chairs. Noting Lussi's interest in the textbook and journal titles, Dr. Daher said, "Ah yes, Dr. Sim, I apologize for the state of my office, but the hospital library is not yet stocked with an adequate range of standard pediatric resources so, meanwhile, I have to bring in my own reference material."

Dr. Daher proved an earnest and concerned listener, nodding frequently as Lussi stressed that there must be an immediate audit to assess deficiencies in the documentation of both patient clinical status and clinical care provided. He seemed eager to comply, but Lussi wished he was a more active participant in the discussion and would offer more suggestions. They agreed that he would designate nursing staff and physicians from Labor and Delivery and the NICU who would work with Lussi and Ann to complete a patient chart audit within the next two-to-three weeks.

When it came to selecting priority educational topics for the physicians, Dr. Daher was far more animated. Two hours later they'd developed a provisional teaching schedule for the next four months. Lussi cautioned that the results of the audit might indicate changes in the order of priority for the topics.

As Lussi drove them back to Children's Hospital, she and Ann shared what they had learned.

"Well, first of all," Ann said, "the NICU Nurse Director's name is Alice Benthal, and she was trained in the UK. We met with ten NICU nurses, all of whom were enthusiastic about the educational program and suggested a list of teaching topics that will fill the schedule for at least six months.

"Alice provided me with a copy of their current in-service teaching schedule. The topics seem appropriate, but there are a lot of cancellations. Alice left the room several times to deal with issues in the NICU, and I noticed that the nurses talked to me more freely about how Labor and Delivery and the NICU function while she was absent. Most notably, there was total consensus that NICU staffing is inadequate. On paper, the staff numbers looked adequate for a level two NICU that has only twelve beds but, according to the nurses, they must attend so many high-risk deliveries that they feel they neglect their patients in the NICU, especially when it comes to writing timely notes in their charts. I must say I'm puzzled by this; why would a level two service have so many high-risk deliveries?"

There was a pause while Lussi took a left turn. "That's fascinating Ann, and it fits with what Dr. Daher told me. He said that the obstetricians expect to perform three thousand deliveries this year. I thought I'd misheard him and asked him to repeat the number. When you think that they are competing with Johns Hopkins Hospital, the University of Maryland Hospital, and several large community hospitals, I can't understand how they can reach anywhere close to that number of annual deliveries. On top of that, the NICU is so small. Even if all three thousand deliveries result from normal pregnancies, they'll have to expect that about forty percent of the babies will have an unpredicted problem that might require care in the NICU. Also, even if each admission is only in the NICU for two days, it will be full almost one hundred percent of the time.

"Dr. Daher also told me that Labor and Delivery service admits high-risk mothers. If they are intending to manage three thousand deliveries, including high-risk pregnancies, they have a grossly inadequate bed capacity in the NICU."

Ann nodded. "Absolutely, Lussi. As a matter of fact, I noticed that they had only one empty bed in the NICU this morning, and there was a severe diabetic in labor and a delivery with a non-reassuring fetal heart tracing going on at the same time. I asked Alice for the total number of NICU nurses in the pool; she told me there were twenty-six. I can't see how this number can cover three shifts per day with vacation and sick time and with the high potential need for one nurse to one patient care for very sick babies, plus coverage of labor and delivery."

"You know Ann, I just can't figure out how the hospital owners got the regulators to OK such mismatched obstetric and NICU capability, especially at a community hospital. How can they run what appears to be a level three obstetric service and provide only level two NICU care? As far as NICU space goes, I wonder if they have a step-down nursery that they didn't show us.

"As soon as we can, we need to look at the range of diagnoses for the high-risk obstetric patients, so that we can tailor the teaching topics to their clinical base and hopefully shed some light on the OB-NICU mismatch."

"Well, one thing they do seem to have plenty of is money," said Ann. "I was very impressed with the equipment in both Labor and Delivery and the NICU, and the hospital is beautiful inside."

After turning onto the grounds of Children's Hospital, Lussi replied. "Yes, I agree, their NICU equipment makes ours look old and shabby, but I wonder if the staff are properly trained to use all of it? I think that this project is going to prove very interesting and challenging for us, Ann. Dr. Daher offered to buy any additional teaching equipment that we require and to provide us with as much space as we need. I'll have to check the terms of our grant to make sure that we can allow them to buy equipment for us. What was your overall impression of Alice Benthal?"

Ann shifted in her seat and replied hesitantly. "She seems knowledgeable about newborn nursing care, at least as far as I could tell in the short time that I was with her. The nurses seem to like her as a person and praised her administrative skills, but they gave me the impression that she's not assertive enough to represent their needs to nursing administration and is dominated by Dr. Daher."

"She did seem a bit submissive when she was with Dr. Daher. I can see why the nurses think he intimidates her." Lussi parked the car.

As they walked into Children's Hospital, Ann smiled broadly. "I can't wait to get started on this program. I can't speak for the physicians, but the nurses really want to learn, and those babies need us."

They had just stepped onto the escalator ascending to the hospital atrium, when Joe Meridian appeared at the top, holding a colorful bouquet of balloons. He proceeded to walk down toward them on the rising elevator, with his arms flung wide and a beaming smile.

A mother with two small boys, just ahead of Lussi and Ann on the escalator, and a teenager on the descending escalator were giggling at Joe's clowning when he declared, "Ah, my two favorite colleagues. You must be returning from South Baltimore Hospital. I can't wait to hear all about your visit."

Now stationary, traveling backward with the ascending escalator, Joe succeeded in distributing balloons to Ann, Lussi, and all three children, before he was deposited back at the top of the escalator.

Chapter 9

Friday, February 6th, 1987, 2:30 p.m.

THREE DAYS AFTER HER RETURN FROM THE FAMILY SKI trip in Norway, Lussi was in her office with Muriel Dressing and the parents of a patient, hearing their complaints regarding the care of their son, Sam, an extremely premature baby who had been a patient in the NICU for almost two months.

"My wife and I take it in in turn to visit Sam, so that one of us is with him for most of the day. When I arrived this morning," said Sam's father, "a nurse I did not recognize was placing a syringe attached to one of Sam's intravenous lines onto a pump. Luckily, Sam has been a patient here for so long that my wife and I are quite familiar with the details of his care. To me, the fluid in the syringe looked like the breast milk my wife expresses for Sam, which I know should be fed into his stomach through a tube in his nose not intravenously. I also know that the only intravenous fluid that looks like milk is the fat solution that you used to give him when he was tiny. I remember you telling us it was a fat solution, Dr. Sim, in one of our early meetings. So, I asked the nurse what was in the syringe, and she told me it was breastmilk. I asked her not to start the pump until I could go to the desk and get someone to come over and check what she was doing. Thankfully, she did what I requested."

Lussi was not offering excuses. "No parent should have to deal with something like this, and I can only offer our empathy and sincere apologies. I would expect an incident like this to undermine your faith in the care we are providing for Sam, and I am willing to arrange for his transfer to another level four NICU in the area and to personally assure you that the cost of the transfer will not be billed to you."

"Oh no, Dr. Sim, we don't want that." Sam's mother said hurriedly. "We feel comfortable with his regular nurses and think Sam has received excellent care up to now."

Sam's father spoke softly. "To tell you the truth, doctor, I *am* finding the thought that I may have arrived just in time to save my son's life extremely unnerving. This episode has shaken both of us badly. We have been so impressed, up to now, by the care Sam has received here and the kindness shown to us by the unit staff.

"I would be ready to disagree with my wife and request Sam's transfer, were it not for the fact that both you and Ms. Dressing have been so open and honest with us. However, if Sam stays in your unit, we need to have your personal assurance that he will only be cared for by regular NICU nurses."

Lussi and Muriel promised that, in the future, no agency nurse would care for Sam and Lussi immediately wrote this order in his patient chart.

After the meeting, Lussi followed Muriel back to her office. Muriel sat down at her desk and Lussi took a seat. They stared at each other until Lussi broke the silence.

"I really admire those parents, Muriel. I don't think I could be as understanding as they are. They are such dedicated visitors already. Now the poor things probably feel obligated to be at Sam's bedside guarding him day and night."

"Believe me, I agree, Lussi," Muriel said with her head in her hands. "How Sam's Dad kept his cool with that nurse I don't know, but she might not have listened to him if he hadn't. I can't believe what's happening in our NICU. On top of it all, I've had two of my best nurses come to me in the past twenty-four hours to give their notice, and I don't blame them. They don't want to work in a grubby NICU that provides sloppy care."

"Muriel, I want so much to get through to the people on the Fifth Floor just how destructive their actions are, but I'm met with a wall of hostility." Hunched in her seat, Lussi sighed. "I feel that I've let you and the patients down because I've built a reputation up there for being confrontational. Once I've got myself wound up to face them, my presentation ends up considerably less than diplomatic. I wish I had the communication skills of someone like Joe Meridian."

"Personally, I prefer people like you who are direct, Lussi. You know where you are with them. Attempting to correct things that need correcting is way better, in my opinion, than doing what a lot of the medical staff do – hide their heads in the sand. Unfortunately, you're frequently left with only the bruises to show for it when you go up against soulless individuals like Sherry Dunstan and Tony Blake."

Lussi looked at her watch, threw back her shoulders, and smiled at Muriel. "Thank you so much for that, Muriel – it was what I needed to hear. I've no right to feel sorry for myself. It's our job to stand up for the patients and this was the last straw."

"Well said Lussi – but watch your back."

"We are going to get the agency nurses out of the NICU, Muriel. Let's get to work on a plan."

Chapter 10

Friday, February 13th, 1987, 11 a.m.

WHEN LUSSI ENTERED SUZANNE SINCLAIR'S OFFICE, FOR what Barbara entered on her schedule as a 'budget review', she was surprised to find Sherry Dunstan sitting there, apparently engaged in a heated verbal exchange with Suzanne. Their dialogue ceased abruptly upon Lussi's arrival. Suzanne waved Lussi to a chair, then nodded in Sherry's direction.

Without preamble, a stone-faced Sherry declared, "There will no longer be agency nurses working in the NICU. Rest assured, Dr. Sim, that Mr. Shultz and I have not made this decision because we have any doubt that, with *adequate* orientation, these agency nurses are quite capable of providing competent care for NICU patients."

I can't believe it – she's shifting the blame onto Ann for their incompetence.

Sherry glanced at Suzanne, who indicated that she should continue. "You have Joe Meridian to thank for this resolution Dr. Sim. The cardiac surgery division has recently received a substantial financial gift from grateful parents. The money is to be put toward building a cardiac research unit. Joe Meridian has talked Christian Carter into assigning a portion of these funds to Nursing. The money will be used to develop a team of nurses who are interested in research to care for all ECMO, cardiology, and cardiac surgery patients in the NICU. Several of our current NICU nurses have already expressed interest.

"This timely addition to the nursing budget will go some way to negate the need to employ agency nurses, however, your division will be expected to contribute additional funds. Ms. Sinclair will provide you with the details."

Sherry stood and stalked out of the office.

As usual, Suzanne was dressed for the runway. Lussi had never seen her in clothing that lacked a designer label. She was a stunningly beautiful woman, with Audrey Hepburn-like features and long, lustrous brunette hair.

"Good morning, Lussi. I apologize for taking you by surprise, but it seems that you have caused quite a stir up here this morning. Mr. Schultz has prior engagements, so he asked me to talk with you and Sherry."

I suspect that Bill delegated this job to me because Sherry is so incensed at Lussi that he didn't think he could handle her. However, for me, witnessing Sherry blowing her top in Bill's office provided a most amusing interlude.

"Yes – well thanks for filling me in, Suzanne. I came expecting to discuss the Division Budget, and I have with me the data sheets you sent me three weeks ago. Do you want to go ahead?"

"Yes, of course, Lussi, but I'm afraid that we now must dispense with the budget I outlined in those spreadsheets. Sherry has informed me that, in addition to the financial contribution from Christian Carter, it will cost your division approximately fifty thousand dollars this year to completely remove the agency nurses from the NICU." Suzanne handed Lussi a two-page document. "Have a look at her numbers – take your time."

Lussi did not dread encounters with Suzanne in the same way she did with Sherry, Bill and Tony Blake.

Despite her rumored infidelity with Bill Shultz, Lussi regarded Suzanne as a highly competent business professional who revealed flashes of humanity when dealing with unpaid patient bills, and open interest in the patients on the rare occasions she visited the NICU. Sherry's data, however, indicated a tough negotiation ahead. Lussi handed the document back to Suzanne, who replaced it with a single sheet.

"Obviously, I have not had the opportunity, yet, to go through her financial data in detail, Lussi, but Sherry's figures look reasonable. The document I just handed you contains my suggestions regarding cuts to your annual budget which would provide the required contribution to Nursing."

"But if I'm interpreting this correctly, Suzanne, the only real choice I have is to reduce my team of neonatologists from four to three and a half positions.?"

"Well, yes, your interpretation might be accurate. Although I am quite open to considering any alternatives you may wish to offer."

Lussi willed herself to remain calm. "Suzanne, I need to remind you that this is a teaching hospital and ours is a large, busy, Level IV NICU. The University has the expectation that our physicians are academically productive, and to achieve this goal they are required to teach and do research, in addition to performing their clinical duties. With a medical staff reduction, even of half a position, there will be insufficient time available to both maintain our university appointments and cover our patient care responsibilities."

Suzanne was about to speak, but Lussi continued. "I should also point out that the research grants awarded to our division bring in significantly more overhead money than is contributed to the hospital by most of the other divisions."

"I do recognize that you run an excellent research program Lussi, but as Bill Shultz has stated repeatedly, the hospital is in a fiscal crisis and, thus, management has the right to demand sacrifices from the staff, which we hope will be temporary. He has made it clear to me that this is not a negotiable issue."

"May I have forty-eight hours to discuss this with my team and get back to you?"

"Yes, of course."

Once Lussi had left, Suzanne sighed and declared to the empty room, "That lady has a spine and genuinely cares about her patients. Sadly, not great survival skills in this business environment."

Back in her own office, Lussi picked abstractedly through her inbox, almost immediately encountering a bright yellow flyer announcing a second town meeting with Bill Schultz. The stated purpose was to present details of a major donation to the Cardiac Surgery division for the development of a state-of-the-art Cardiac Research Center.

Lussi made a mental note to thank Joe Meridian when she next saw him and mused over the possible identity of the parents making what must be a sizeable donation. Families with this level of financial means were not common in the immediate hospital service area, but cardiac surgery patients were admitted from all over the United States and from other countries, so the families of their patients were frequently financially well to do.

Lussi picked up the phone. "Hi Barbara, would you set up a meeting for me with the other neonatologists? Preferably Monday afternoon and no later than the day after. Tell them that it is to discuss an important, confidential matter that has just arisen."

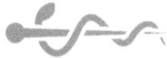

7:45 p.m.

SUZANNE WAS IN A REFLECTIVE MOOD AS SHE NURSED A cocktail and waited for her husband in the bar of a restaurant in Baltimore Harbor. It was unusual for George to be late, especially since they were meeting to celebrate Valentine's Day early because tomorrow George would be out of town on business.

George was the youngest of three sons. Born and raised in Texas, his father opened a small swimming pool company in the early 1950s, with his two older sons. By the mid-1960s, the company was highly regarded as a local purveyor of quality swimming pools.

George had joined the pool company in the 1960s, after following his muse for a while as a drummer in a rock band. He'd told Suzanne that he quickly realized that he wasn't cut out for the construction side of things but discovered an interest in designing pools and the area around them. He loved the challenge of transforming a plain backyard into a stunning oasis while keeping costs reasonable by enhancing preexisting features and natural resources, using his innovative skills to cope with challenging topography. George designed pools with artistic curves and creatively located deep and shallow areas, surrounded by a relaxing sanctuary.

Designs by George were in such high demand that, by the mid-nineteen seventies, the pool firm had made an initial public offering and Suzanne was impressed by how well their stock had performed since then. There were now branches of the company in all major cities in the United

States and smaller outlets in most towns with populations over one hundred thousand. His older brothers had both retired, and George had taken over as CEO.

George was married to his first wife for thirty-two years. Two years after she died of cancer, Suzanne entered his life and found it incredibly easy to sweep him off his feet. George was significantly older than her and no Adonis, but over time and against her calculations she'd been captivated by his integrity, modesty, generosity, and adoration. She characterized her feelings for George as profound fondness; complicated by concealed remorse for the instances when she was not living up to his image of her.

Suzanne was aware that George had also fallen in love with Baltimore City, long before he and she moved from Texas to Howard County, Maryland. In fact, he would have been happy to live downtown full-time had she not made it clear that she wanted to build a sizeable stable. Instead, he'd purchased a condominium with a view across the Baltimore harbor, that he and Suzanne used when they had social events in the city or had to work late.

George approached from behind and kissed her on the cheek. "Hello, darling; so sorry I'm late. The Town Planning meeting adjourned almost half an hour late."

Suzanne glanced up from her fixed gaze into the glowing fireplace and smiled impishly at George. She had chosen to sit as far as possible from the bar, beside the fireplace in a dimly lit corner of the room. She very much disliked being in a bar alone and found that the best way to avoid unwanted attention was to strictly avoid eye contact.

"Hi, George dear. Was there any roughhousing at the meeting?"

George laughed and placed his beer on the table, removed his coat, and slung it over the back of his chair. "No, everyone was well-behaved – just more bad news about industry leaving the city. How about you, darling – did you have a good day?"

"Nothing out of the usual. Just the peasants revolting again."

"Aren't the 'peasants', as you call them, ever justified in rebelling, Suzanne? From what you've told me and from reading the newspaper, Children's Hospital would seem to be a stressful, authoritarian place to work."

Suzanne laughed and rolled her eyes. "George Sinclair, I swear you are a communist in capitalist clothing."

Just then the Maître d' appeared. Picking up their drinks, they followed him into the dining room.

Chapter 11

Wednesday, February 18th, 1987, 8:30 a.m.

LUSSI FELT REJUVENATED AS SHE DROVE TO SOUTH BALtimore Community Hospital. Her colleagues had agreed to donate, by taking a reduction in pay, the remaining fifty thousand dollars required to replace the agency nurses. Lussi, being the highest paid, would take the most substantial cut; the residual amount would be split between the other three neonatologists based on their seniority. Once Lussi's team had corroborated, in a closed-door meeting with Suzanne, that Lussi had placed no pressure on them to approve this plan, Suzanne expressed no opposition.

Lussi was also eager to inspect what Dr. Daher had told her were unused rooms available to her outreach teaching program on the South Baltimore Hospital Campus. Outside the NICU it is a little-known fact that the upper airway of an adult ferret anatomically matches the airway of a premature human baby, but inside the field of neonatal healthcare education, ferrets provide an excellent model for teaching health professionals how to place an airway tube in a small premature baby.

Ann Castle kept the ferrets at her home as pets. Each animal had a name and, to maintain their acceptability in human company, she bathed them frequently. However, animals were not allowed in the hospital, so before Lussi and Ann could set up teaching workshops, they must locate space outside the main hospital building. At many hospitals it was not easy to find suitable space, however, Dr. Daher thought he might have found the perfect location.

On entering the NICU, Lussi found Dr. Daher dressed in scrubs, placing umbilical lines in a patient.

He looked up and smiled when Lussi said, "Hi Naeem, thanks so much for arranging this visit to Building C."

"I'm sorry that I can't go with you right now, Lussi, but I will join you there when I've got these lines in. In the pocket of my white coat, hanging in the scrub room, you will find a key ring with four keys on it. The one you need is labeled Building C, which is behind the hospital – you'll see signs outside the main entrance of the hospital directing you there. The building houses some office space and three sizeable multipurpose rooms. Why don't you go ahead and look at them and I'll catch up with you?"

After a short walk to the rear of the main hospital, Lussi arrived at the entrance to Building C. On the delivery dock fronting Building B, next door, were four men unloading two large delivery trucks. Otherwise, the area was deserted.

Once inside, Lussi located the three empty rooms described by Dr. Daher without difficulty. The space was, in fact, one large room that could be converted into three smaller rooms using folding partitions suspended from the ceiling. The space would be perfect for the teaching workshops.

Dr. Daher had not yet joined her, so Lussi decided to explore. Only an intermittent low hum and vibration from the heating system broke the silence. Lussi was amazed that so much space was vacant. They never seemed to have enough at Children's.

There were three small offices, furnished but obviously not in current use, and a kitchen. Opposite the kitchen door, on the other side of the hallway, a double metal door bore a large red STOP sign and the message *Authorized Personnel Only*. There was a keypad on the wall to the right of the door.

What on earth? This is odd.

It was not the door itself that was remarkable – it was the infant transport incubator and ventilator that stood in front of it. There was lukewarm water in the humidifier on the ventilator and, judging by the damp areas and three spots of fresh blood on the mattress, the incubator had recently been occupied.

Dr. Daher assured me that this is not a patient care building, so what is this equipment doing here?

Intrigued and eager to question Naeem Daher, Lussi returned to the hospital.

In the NICU, she found an apologetic Naeem removing his gloves and gown. "The X-ray showed the venous line had deviated into the liver, Lussi, so I had to reposition it. Sorry, I didn't make it over. What do you think of the space in Building C?"

"The space is perfect, Naeem. Thank you so much for finding it for me."

Lussi paused, to carefully choose her next words. "However, I'm a little puzzled by some recently used newborn transport equipment I came across outside a restricted access door in the building. Why would it be left in a building not used for patient care, Naeem?"

The color drained from Naeem's face and Lussi thought he looked scared. "Are you okay, Naeem?"

Although still towering above Lucy, Dr. Daher seemed to have shrunk in stature. He stuttered, "Oh, yes, yes, of course, Lussi – animal research, I believe on dogs, is done in the research labs in building D, and I believe the door you are describing connects with the research building.

However, it is not permitted to move research equipment or research animals out of the lab. Thank you for letting me know about this, I will follow up."

Lussi smiled to disguise her disbelief of Naeem's explanation. *What is an animal research facility doing in a community hospital? Such laboratories are usually located in university hospitals or large inner-city hospitals linked to a medical school. What type of research animal would be a good fit for a newborn incubator – a puppy or a piglet, maybe, but certainly not an average-sized dog.*

Rather than voicing her questions, Lussi continued to smile. "That's exciting information, Naeem. I have grant funding to do an animal study at Children's, but there's currently no lab space available there. I've been waiting for over six months and could end up losing the grant if I don't find space soon. You'd be doing me a huge favor if you would give me the name and telephone number of the head of the research laboratories. If I could get space here, that would be wonderful. In return, this hospital would receive the overhead money that the grant pays and the kudos for housing the study."

Naeem's persisting pallor indicated that Lussi's enthusiasm had done little to alleviate his distress. "Well Lussi, you know, it isn't a very large research unit and I doubt…"

Lussi interrupted, "Naeem, take time to consider what a great opportunity this would be for you to gain research experience and enhance your curriculum vitae. Plus, you will have helped to bring a significant amount of money into the research labs; the overheads for my study are close to three million dollars over five years. May I inform the research director of your interest and include you in my list of investigators?"

"It's generous of you, Lussi, to consider including me in your research. I did some clinical research during my training in neonatology, but I've never done animal research. Wouldn't that be a problem?"

"No, not at all, Naeem. I always have at least one of our fellows working with me in the lab, and most of them have never done any research before. My animal model is quite easy to set up and you are welcome to work with me on that part of the study, or there's a purely clinical component that might interest you more. I'll get you a copy of the protocol, and you can let me know what you think. I would be happy to have you as a co-investigator."

Hesitant and obviously avoiding eye contact, Naeem produced the telephone number for the Director of Research Laboratories, Dr. Paul Kader.

On the drive back to Children's Hospital, Lussi ruminated on unanswered questions arising from the ongoing audits of patient admissions to the NICU and Obstetrics services at South Baltimore Hospital. The audits were progressing more slowly than she would like, but even at this early stage, it was clear that the Obstetric data were not matching up with the NICU data when it came to certain diagnostic categories. Since the beginning of the year, for example, the high-risk obstetric service at South Baltimore had accepted three maternal transfers from out-of-state hospitals that Lussi did not recognize, all with the generic diagnosis of *Fetal Cardiac Anomaly*. However, over the same period, there were no infants admitted to their NICU with diagnoses that fit this category.

If all three fetal heart anomalies were lethal it would explain why none of the babies were admitted to the NICU. However, if this was the case, what was the indication for interstate in-utero transport? The mother could decide on abortion versus spontaneous delivery at her local hospital.

If they were treatable anomalies, these mothers should have been transported to a major medical center in the first place, rather than a local community hospital. The diagnosis of fetal anomaly indicated that the mother was not the primary patient – however, her fetus would require immediate, highly sophisticated emergency care either in-utero or immediately after delivery, at an institution with a level three or four NICU. Dr. Daher assures me that the level two NICU that he directs is the only one at South Baltimore Hospital.

It also puzzles me that Christian Carter is consulting at South Baltimore – why do they need a pediatric cardiac surgeon? Perhaps he only does diagnostic consultations? Of course, he is also trained in adult cardiac surgery, so he could consult on all age groups and provide advice – but he can't do surgery at South Baltimore Hospital, and he would surely refer infants with treatable heart conditions to himself at Children's Hospital. Even though he can't do heart transplants he can still perform all the other surgical procedures, but I am certain that none of the three mothers admitted to South Baltimore Hospital with a diagnosis of fetal cardiac anomaly produced infants who were then transferred to our NICU at Children's.

Something isn't as it should be.

As soon as she arrived back in her office at Children's, Lussi called the number supplied by Naeem Daher. The male secretary, who answered the phone with a pronounced Irish accent, was accommodating, although he emphasized more than once that the director was an extremely busy man. When Lussi stressed that the meeting was urgent and involved a large research grant with significant overhead financing, he found her a thirty-minute opening, five days hence, to meet with Paul Kader, Ph.D., at his office in the Research Building.

Chapter 12

Monday, February 23rd, 1987, 2:50 p.m.

WEDGED BETWEEN THE REAR OF THE HOSPITAL AND Building C, the unassuming entrance to Research Building D formed a peak, on what Lussi gathered from the roof lines must be a triangular structure.

To the left of the entrance was a small brass plate listing four names, each with a separate push button; Lussi pressed the button labeled P. Kader, Ph.D. Dr. Kader's Irish secretary announced through the intercom that he would be there immediately to let her in. Four minutes later Lussi was sitting in the waiting room outside Paul Kader's office.

Immediately upon entering the building, it became clear to Lussi that it was indeed wedge-shaped, widening from the entrance with progressively deviating corridors forming the left and right sides of the triangle. Between the corridors, directly opposite the entrance, were the glass double doors of Dr. Kader's office suite. The waiting room, which retained the triangular shape, had windows facing onto the corridors on both sides. The plush carpeting and expensive modern decoration struck Lussi as unlike anything she'd encountered in the research laboratories she'd worked in.

The far wall of the waiting room formed the hypotenuse. At the left end was a sizeable workspace for the secretary, to the right of which was a door with a sign indicating Dr. Paul

Kader's office. On the wall to the right of this door hung a large plan of the interior of the building.

Dr. Kader having not yet returned from an outside meeting, Lussi walked over to examine the plan. It was clear that the triangular form persisted the full length of the building, with six laboratories – three on each side of the center of the triangle. The two largest and most distant laboratories formed the base of the triangle; on the left of the midline was Cardiovascular Dynamics and on the right was the Animal Facility.

Interrupted in her study by the appearance of Dr. Kader at her side, Lussi turned with a smile.

He extended his hand and, with a perfect upper-class English accent, said, "I must apologize profusely for keeping you waiting, Dr. Sim. As you yourself have had the opportunity to observe, the traffic on the beltway today is abominable."

Lussi shook his hand, "Thank you for fitting me in, Dr. Kader; I know your time is limited." She was immediately struck by both his accent and his height, which she estimated at over six feet six inches. He was handsome, dark-skinned, bearded, and immaculately dressed in what looked to Lussi like a silk suit. His was a very different style of dress from even the most distinguished male researchers she had previously encountered, all of whom habitually dressed for work in an open-neck shirt and jeans.

Inside Paul Kader's spacious office, there were no windows. The furnishings were lavish and there was expensive-looking artwork on the walls and on shelves, but not a single textbook or journal. Dr. Kader waved Lussi to a comfortable leather armchair next to an octagonal, inlaid, white marble table and took the chair opposite her.

Lussi openly admired the table as she took her seat. "I see that you have excellent taste, Dr. Sim," Kader remarked. "This table is made of the same marble used to build the Taj Mahal and, like the Taj Mahal, it is inlaid with semi-precious stones. Would you care for a cup of coffee or tea?"

"Oh, thank you no, Dr. Kader, I'm fine. Your table is exquisite. Did you receive the material I FedEx'd to you?"

"Yes indeed, and I have reviewed it with care. I find your hypothesis intriguing and the piglet model you have developed impressive, Dr. Sim. You have a notable research track record, especially considering that your medical school was not in the United States. I know from first-hand experience how difficult it can be for immigrant physicians to obtain research grants in this country."

"Well, I was lucky enough to be recommended by one of my professors in Norway to an excellent research mentor in this country. That has helped me to gain recognition from funding agencies relatively quickly. I know your labs have not been operating for long. Has your animal facility previously cared for pigs?"

"No, to date our animals have all been dogs, however, I don't foresee any problem dealing with pigs, especially of the small size that you study. Your research protocol outlines the feeding and other care requirements in detail. I shared it with our animal technicians, and they feel that they are fully equipped to provide the maintenance that your study animals require."

"That sounds great, Dr. Kader. May I tour the available laboratory space and the animal facility after this meeting?"

"Well, Dr. Sim," Kader leaned back in his chair and looked at his watch, "Since this unit opened only recently, we are very interested in attracting quality researchers such as yourself, and" he smiled, "the overhead funding would also be useful. Regrettably, I have another meeting scheduled in five minutes, but I can tell you that I am certain that the resources here, including the animal facility, will suit your project perfectly. However, before I go further, I must confer with the members of my Research Board and obtain their approval. I'll get back to you as soon as I can and, if the Board agrees, I'll arrange for you to see the laboratories."

As she rose to leave, Lussi hoped her disappointment did not show on her face. She thanked Dr. Kader, and they again shook hands.

Just before reaching the office door, Lussi turned and asked, "What is your own primary area of research interest, Dr. Kader? What type of dogs do you use?"

Kader was, Lussi thought, rather pointedly absorbed in sorting through the pile of papers on his desk. He looked up at her with raised eyebrows, as if surprised by her question.

"Cardiovascular – of course in adult dogs. If you would excuse me – I really do have to run, Dr. Sim."

Lussi needed to see more of the building. Despite Paul Kader's pleasant manner and stated admiration of her research achievements, she felt uncomfortable. Nothing about Kader or his office suite was compatible with a medical research facility. And then there was his incredibly generic response to her question about his research field. Needing an excuse not to leave the building immediately, Lussi asked Kader's secretary for directions to the ladies' restroom.

Turning left outside the entrance to the office suite, as instructed, Lussi followed the corridor toward the rear of the building. She could see through the frosted glass windows in the laboratory doors that lights were on in the two laboratories that she passed on her way to the restroom.

Outside each lab, to the right of the door, was an emergency decontamination shower. The opposite wall of the corridor was windowless and devoid of decoration. The silence felt ominous, and the place seemed to be deserted.

The women's restroom appeared unremarkable, with six stalls. Lussi was about to leave when she noticed what looked like the wrist of a surgical gown, overhanging the opening of one of the circular trash cans built into the counter. As she gingerly pulled the gown from the can, a pair of bloody surgical gloves fell out of the folds.

Why would anyone dispose of a contaminated surgical gown and gloves in a trash bin in the ladies' room? That is negligence. Having stuffed the gown and gloves back into the trash receptacle and washed her hands, Lussi left the restroom and continued down the corridor.

As Lussi had learned from the plan on the wall of Kader's office suite, the animal facility was the laboratory furthest from the office suite that was accessible from this corridor. There were two entrances, each with its own decontamination shower, however, although bright light shone through the windows in both doors, there were no outward signs of activity. Lucci had not tried the doors of the other laboratories for fear of being caught, but by now she was emboldened by her persistent failure to detect human activity. Both doors were locked.

The hallway ended abruptly at a wall.

How do you cross over to the corridor on the other side of the building from here? There must be an internal door between the animal facility and the cardiovascular dynamics lab on the other side.

The only decoration in the entire corridor adorned the wall in front of her; a large, framed print of two bulls locking horns. One of the bulls had lost the tip of a horn, which was bleeding profusely. *Who would have the poor taste to hang a picture like this outside an animal care facility? And the silence – there doesn't appear to be anybody or any animals around. Kader implied there was research involving dogs currently ongoing, but this place doesn't smell or sound like an animal facility.*

Lussi retraced her steps to the restroom. She searched the room for something, anything, that might relate to the contaminated surgical gown. Scanning the room for signage, or other helpful information, Lussi's attention focused on the stall furthest from the entrance, which was clearly larger than the others. According to a sign on this door, on the other side was an infant changing room, however, the door was locked, and, unlike the other stalls, there was no door handle or any other visible means of opening it.

This is unexpected – I've never worked in an animal research facility that allowed children inside, even the offspring of employees.

The doors and side walls of the stalls extended all the way to the floor, but the space between the tops of the doors and the ceiling was generous.

My kingdom for a stepladder.

A few seconds later Lussi was removing the tall metal canister from a trash receptacle. She placed the canister upside down outside the changing room. Standing on it, she was able to see over the top of the door.

No handle or lock was visible on the inside of the door. The stall contained a hinged shelf for diaper changing on the left wall, and on the far wall were a toilet and sink. The right-hand wall of the stall did not extend all the way to the rear; there was an opening to the right of the sink.

Although Lussi was on the alert for someone entering, there continued to be no signs of life in the corridor. Pondering how to gain access to the changing room, Lussi scrutinized the entire bathroom.

There were five sinks cut into the counter. On the wall behind each sink was an imposing mirror, dotted around the borders with small circular lights. Lussi stood back and stared at the row of mirrors.

They look incongruous. Obviously expensive mirrors with high-tech lighting, in a bathroom that is otherwise utilitarian, with linoleum flooring and laminate countertops. And why install mirrors with individual lighting when the ceiling lights are more than adequate?

Lussi used the wall switch near the restroom entrance to turn the ceiling lights off and on. The lights around all the mirrors turned off and on in unison with the ceiling lights. However, despite their coordinated response to the main light switch, Lussi noted a white push button in the right lower corner of each mirror.

Hmmm, more overkill. Those must be independent switches for the lights on each mirror.

With the ceiling lights on, Lussi pressed the button on the mirror closest to the restroom entrance and turned off only the lighted circles on this mirror. She then pressed the button several more times, with the expected results.

Well, that was a long shot, but there is nothing else in here that seems so out of place.

Lussi stood back and exhaled noisily through pursed lips while she again studied the row of mirrors.

Hold on a minute – that is interesting.

The button on the mirror closest to the changing room was in the same position as the button on the other four.

However, unlike their pristine white buttons, the button on this one showed wear and discoloration and, surrounding it on the mirror, were multiple fingerprints. Lussi pressed this button and the lights around the mirror turned off, as expected. She pushed it again and the mirror lights came on. The third push turned the mirror lights off once more. Driven more by frustration than hope, Lussi pressed the button for the fourth time, and, to her astonishment, the door of the changing room swung open.

Positioning the trash canister to prevent the door from closing behind her, Lussi walked over to the opening in the far right-hand corner of the changing room. In front of her was a short corridor, ending at the doors of an elevator.

Lussi looked at her watch. It was four twenty, p.m. She was not expected to return to Children's today and she'd told Rachel and John that she would be home about six p.m. Now was not the time to stop.

Then Lussi remembered her pager was still on. *I can't stop now, there is something underhanded going on here. I hate to be out of contact, but I can't risk my pager going off. I'm certain I'm on the verge of discovering something of vital importance. I must continue for a little, while my luck holds.*

Lussi turned off her pager and pressed the call button for the elevator. Inside there were buttons for the ground floor, basement, and first floor. She pressed the button for the first floor.

Stepping out of the elevator, Lussi found herself facing a bank of green metal lockers. She heard female voices in the distance, and behind the lockers she found shelves loaded with surgical gowns, scrub suits, head and shoe covers, and gloves. She was in a surgical changing room.

Locating an empty locker, Lussi exchanged her outer clothes for a scrub suit. She put on a head cover, mask, and shoe covers, scrubbed her hands and forearms for three minutes, and then, using full sterile technique, put on a gown and gloves. She emerged from behind the rows of lockers and walked purposefully through the automatic doors on the far side of the scrub room. Two women seated on a bench talking animatedly paid no attention to her. Turning to her right, a few steps brought her to a second automatic door with a sign above it announcing the Cardiac ICU.

Once through this door, Lussi was assailed by the familiar mechanical sounds of a NICU; ventilators hissing and monitors beeping. The light in her immediate surroundings was subdued, but a few feet ahead far brighter light emanated from below. Passing the entrances to narrow passages on her right and left, Lussi arrived at the top of a stair leading down to a large, circular room holding eight infant warmer stations arranged in a circle. Ringing each warmer station were small floodlights embedded in the floor.

Lussi noted that four of the warmers were empty; the remainder were occupied by small infants. Each infant was attended by a masked individual wearing a scrub suit. From where Lussi stood, she could see that the shadowy walkways on either side of her ultimately merged, to completely circle the room below and, with minimal risk of discovery, provide a clear view from above of each warmer station.

Lussi entered the walkway to her left, which proved sufficiently narrow to allow her a direct view of the patients below even with her back pressed against the wall. The infant on the first occupied warmer was receiving pump feeds through a tube inserted through his nose; there were three intravenous lines running. This infant was motionless, with pale grey skin color, and the breathing rate set for the ventilator was high. Lussi pushed her back harder against the corridor wall as an X-ray technician pushing a mobile X-ray machine entered the room below, stopping at this infant's warmer and, after exchanging a few words with the attendant, proceeding to set up her machine. Once the technician's attention was absorbed in the process of taking X-rays, Lussi felt it was safe to move on.

On the next warmer was an infant who appeared to have undergone a recent major surgical procedure to the left chest, based on the fresh incision extending the length of the sternum. A tube, draining bloody fluid into a chest drain system, was in place to the left of the incision. This infant was also on a ventilator and appeared to be heavily sedated. An attendant was hanging blood for transfusion.

Lussi could hardly contain her shock and confusion. *Why is a unit caring for critically ill infants apparently operating covertly?*

On the third warmer, a surprisingly healthy-looking infant sucked a pacifier and, despite the restraints in place around ankles and wrists, wriggled actively. Next to the warmer was an empty incubator into which, it appeared, the attendant was preparing to transfer the baby.

On arrival above the fourth occupied warmer Lussi was flabbergasted. She would have recognized Oliver Turner anywhere. Supposedly dead, here he was, receiving oxygen through small cannulas in his nostrils while actively moving his arms and legs. His color was good, and he was focusing on the face of his attendant and smiling, just like any other two-month-old infant.

I've got to get out of here and get help.

Edging to her right, Lussi returned to the top of the stairs down to the NICU. As she was turning away from the stairs, into the main corridor which would take her back to the scrub room, something substantial hit her on the head and left shoulder from behind.

Despite her agony, Lussi twisted her body and grabbed at a shadowy outline behind her, attempting to drag her assailant down with her as she fell.

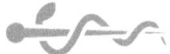

6:35 p.m.

Curled up on the sofa in the family room, Rachel was working on her homework, John was in the kitchen making himself a pre-dinner peanut butter and jelly sandwich next to Howard, who was on the phone ordering takeout pizza.

As soon as he hung up the phone, Howard said, "John, I'm going to call Mom to find out how much longer she will be. Would you tell your sister the pizza will be here in twenty minutes?"

Howard double-checked Lussi's schedule hanging inside the pantry door. He then called the Children's Hospital switchboard, but Lussi did not answer the phone in her office or respond to three attempts to page her. Next, he asked the switchboard to page the neonatologist on night call. Dr. Mary Morrison promptly answered her pager. She was in her office getting ready to go home and offered to look on Barbara Melnick's desk for details of Lussi's schedule that day.

"Howard, Lussi was in her office this morning before I went to the NICU for rounds. Looking at her schedule, she apparently had an appointment with Dr. Kader at three p.m. this afternoon, but it doesn't say where. I'm pretty sure there isn't a Dr. Kader here at Children's. Has she mentioned this person to you?"

"I know Lussi had a meeting set up with some research guy at South Baltimore Community Hospital today, but I don't recall her mentioning his name. It is very unlike her not to respond to her pager. Maybe she's stuck in traffic on the beltway."

"Yes, of course, Howard, she would have to take the beltway to drive home from there. It is also possible that Lussi returned to her office after the appointment, but I was busy with an emergency in the NICU, and I didn't get back to the office suite until about twenty minutes ago. There's nothing scheduled for Lussi after the South Baltimore appointment."

"Lussi is always so conscientious about staying in contact, Mary. I'm thinking back to the abduction from the hospital garage and hoping that I'm crazy to imagine something like that happening again."

"Maybe her pager isn't working, Howard? I'm going to try paging her on the overhead system and I'll ask Security to search the hospital and parking garage. I'll call you back as soon as I know anything more."

Over eight hours and multiple phone calls later, Howard, Rachel, and John were asleep in chairs in the family room, close to the telephone.

Chapter 13

Tuesday, February 24th, 1987, 6:45 a.m.

Suzanne Sinclair felt tense – a rare sensation for her. Not only had Bill Schultz left for work early and deputized his wife to notify her that he would not be picking her up, but Lussi Sim was making waves.

What is Bill up to? I can't afford interruptions in my information flow right now.

As she prepared breakfast, Suzanne attempted to hide her stress from George, however, she momentarily lost control when a jug of orange juice slipped from her grasp and shattered on the kitchen floor. Verbalizing her thoughts, she exclaimed, "Damn that Sim woman. She's probably been interfering again in something that isn't her business."

George put down his newspaper and said gently, "I know you don't mean that, darling. You've told me several times that you like her."

"Oh, for God's sake George, must you always be so saintly?"

"Saintly? Not on your life, my dear. Much more fun to have some flaws."

Suzanne looked at George and, despite herself, burst out laughing.

The phone rang and George picked it up. "Hello. Yes, you've just caught her." George handed the receiver to Suzanne. "It's Dr. Sim's husband."

"Hello, Ms. Sinclair, Howard Sim here. I apologize for the early call. Last night I reported to the Baltimore police that my wife is missing. They were unconvinced initially – said it was too early to launch a search, but her designation as a Missing Person is now official. I've tried several times to contact Mr. Schultz at the hospital but was informed that he has not arrived yet and that the hospital does not provide home phone numbers. Luckily, my daughter remembered that my wife and she bumped into you and your husband at the hospital a few weeks ago. She was impressed because your husband treated her as an adult. When she said she was interested in photography, he gave her his business card with your home number on it."

"I have been notified of your wife's disappearance and the police involvement, Howard. What can I do to help?"

"The police have asked me to provide contact information for Lussi's colleagues. I understand that to give out this information, the switchboard needs the permission of a senior hospital executive."

Suzanne had a file in her home office that contained work and home phone numbers for all the medical staff at Children's Hospital, but she simply did not have time to deal with this. She was already running late.

"I'm happy to supply you with the information you require, Howard, and will call the switchboard now and inform them that it is OK for you to call your wife's colleagues. I'm late for work. Do you mind if I delegate my husband to help you with the phone numbers?"

"Not at all, Ms. Sinclair. That is kind of him."

"Hold on while I get the file."

Suzanne retrieved the file from her office, relocking the door behind her.

Handing the file to George, she said, "George I'm really pressed for time, and Howard Sim urgently requires the home phone numbers for staff in the neonatology division. He is holding on the kitchen phone."

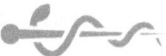

6:46 a.m.

LUSSI COULD NOT MOVE AND HAD NEVER FELT SO COLD. She sensed a velvet blackness enfolding her. As she slipped in and out of consciousness, she became aware of a figure materializing from the blackness. She tried to call out and, although she could not form the words, the figure seemed to hear her. But the eyes that turned on her fleetingly were blazing with fury, and blood vessels filled to bursting bulged from his forehead.

She heard something shatter. Then shouting and screaming. Lussi knew her brothers and sister would be huddled under their bed-clothes and she, as the eldest, must leave the safety of her velvet cavern to intervene downstairs. Why could she not compel her body to follow orders?

Gradually, Lussi comprehended that rather than in a bed from her childhood, she was lying, head uppermost, on a sloping surface. There was a severe, throbbing pain in her head and left shoulder. When she opened her eyes, the darkness persisted. The sounds of violence had now been replaced by loud, furious buzzing.

As sensation returned to her fingertips, Lussi could feel the gritty surface she was lying on. There was a strong aroma that reminded her of cookies just beginning to burn.

It seemed like hours before Lussi was able to move her arms and legs sufficiently to roll onto her stomach, discovering as she did so that the surface on which she was lying was highly abrasive and that she was dressed only in her underwear and shoes. The skin on her elbows and knees suffered the most, but she wasn't certain which was more excruciating, the pain in her head, shoulder, elbows, and knees, or the deafening buzzing echoing around her. Small flying objects were constantly colliding with her.

Despite the protests from her body, Lussi refused to lie still. She stretched out both arms horizontally and, rolling from side to side, was able to touch low metal walls on both sides of her. She concluded that she was lying on a gutter-shaped ramp. She inferred from the reverberating echo when she shouted for help that the ramp was in a cavernous space. The echo of the buzzing also indicated that it originated from her surroundings, rather than inside her head.

By now, Lussi's memory was returning. The discovery of Oliver Turner in the concealed NICU. *Someone hit me. Am I still at South Baltimore Hospital? I'm obviously in danger – unless whoever hit me thinks I'm dead.*

Ignoring the pain, Lussi forced herself onto her hands and knees. She began to edge backward in a bear-like posture, down the steep slope. She dug her feet into the grit and tried to keep her abraded knees above the surface. Now that she'd begun to sweat, the grit grew sticky and flayed the palms of her hands. She had to stop frequently to rest and thanked her lucky stars she still had her shoes.

Without warning, there was a thunderous rattling and the surface beneath Lussi lurched into motion, throwing her off her hands and knees. Now helpless, flat on her stomach on a moving ramp, she was rapidly carried backward and downward. Grit was entering her mouth, nostrils, and eyes as she endeavored to keep her head raised.

Suddenly, the surface below her disappeared and she was ejected into open space. Instinctively, she arched backward and flung out her arms and legs, attempting to slow her velocity; a trick she learned as a child in Oslo, jumping into snow drifts from the garage roof.

Lussi landed head down, face up, once again sliding fast down a slope. All around her was falling grit which, to her amazement, she could now see in a dim grey light when she dared to open her eyes. She came to a stop, her back skinned by friction and her head embedded in gluey grit. Strangely, the grit that clogged her mouth tasted pleasantly sweet. She was able to free her arms and clear a little of it from her eyes and nose. Her eyes were running and throbbing, nevertheless, she could dimly see a huge metal cone high above her, spewing an avalanche of what she now realized was raw sugar. Hovering around her were legions of bees. Lussi reckoned she'd been stung numerous times during her descent.

Rotating back onto her hands and knees, Lussi crawled the short distance to the foot of the sugar mountain and then kept going until she encountered areas of relatively bare concrete floor.

Now out of immediate danger from the falling sugar, Lussi was able to think more clearly. She recalled touring the Domino Sugar factory about six months previously, with an invited group of physicians and nutritionists. She was almost certain that she was now inside the huge hangar near the dock that housed raw sugar delivered by ship from all over the world. Their tour guide, she remembered, had informed the group that each mountain of sugar in the hangar was at least sixty feet high.

I'm lucky to be alive.

Lussi looked around her. Daylight was now entering the hangar through the conveyor belt aperture above her. There were no windows in the hangar, but from the wall nearest to her light filtered through the narrow slats of a louvered air vent. As the sun rose, she was able to make out, in the sugar littering the floor, oversized tire tracks and dead bees. She could also now distinguish, through the sugar dust in the air, at least four saccharine mountains.

There was a wide opening in the wall closest to Lussi, through which she could also see daylight. This led to a dingy stairwell, coated with industrial grime. She was separated from a descending metal staircase by a floor-to-ceiling chain link barrier with a padlocked gate. The source of light was a grimy glass window in the frustratingly inaccessible exit door visible at the foot of the metal staircase.

Her watch was missing. However, Lussi figured that, if this was a weekday, it would not be long after dawn that workers would start arriving in the hangar. Would her captors be among them? Whoever put her on the conveyor belt obviously had some knowledge of the workings of the sugar hangar, but they did not appear to know what time the conveyor belt would shut down for the day, something that surely a regular employee would know.

One thing of which Lussi was certain – her captors had intended her burial in the mountain of sugar before she regained consciousness. She couldn't take the risk of an unwitting encounter with them. She had to find a way out of the hangar without drawing the attention of the work crew. This wasn't going to be simple, clad as she was in only her brassiere and underpants, and covered head-to-toe in abrasions, bee stings, and bloodstained sugar.

The only details about the hangar building that Lussi could remember from her tour were that it was rectangular, and the loading bay for vehicles was at the opposite end from the dock where the ships unloaded the sugar. But she had no idea where she was now in relation to the loading bay. She set off limping slowly along the wall to her right, shortly encountering a row of doors, numbered from one to four, all of which were locked. A large clock on the wall at the far end of the row told her that it was twenty-two minutes past seven. Below the clock was a fifth door, labeled *Toilet*. This door was not locked.

While removing as much of the sugar and blood from her body as she could, Lussi reviewed her options. It seemed likely that some members of the Children's Hospital's upper management were involved in whatever was going on at South Baltimore, so going to the police might be tricky, even if they did believe her. Though, what alternatives did she have?

Ann Castle! She lives less than a mile from the sugar factory, on Federal Hill. If I could make it to her house by eight-fifteen a.m. I might catch Ann before she leaves for work.

After a quick wash, and with a viable escape plan under development, Lussi felt revitalized and more able to face the pain she experienced with every step.

Maybe I can find something to wrap myself in; would a place like this have fire blankets? I must get close to the loading bay doors so that I can stay in the shadows and choose a time to slip through as soon as they open.

The far wall of the hangar was now visible, and Lussi thought she could see the loading bay doors delineated by a slim outline of daylight. As she made her way toward the doors, she was overjoyed to encounter several yellow reflective jackets hanging on a row of wall hooks. She chose a large one. The more of herself she could hide inside it, the better. She put on the jacket and pulled up the collar.

Minutes after she reached the loading bay doors, they began to slide open. Lussi pushed herself back into the shadows. The doors stopped moving, leaving about a three-foot overlap beyond the hangar wall on both sides. Lussi crept sideways and peered around the door. Outside was a wide alley, shadowed by a huge multistory red brick building opposite her which had seen better days. There were multiple missing and broken windows, the paint had almost disappeared from doors and windows, and the building was caked with dirt and rust.

The concrete surface of the alley was marked by interlacing tire tracks; however, it was empty except for a large yellow loader parked to her left. To her right, the alley dead-ended at another red brick building with a tall, white chimney. Piles of sugar were scattered around the loading dock.

The cargo ship would be docked at the other end of the hangar so, once outside, Lussi would remain invisible to the crew unloading the sugar. She couldn't help envisaging her corpse falling out of the loader bucket but, quickly erasing this image, she slipped outside.

About thirty yards to her right, a figure in orange overalls, whom she hadn't seen from inside the hangar, was leaning against a wall smoking a cigarette. She waved, hoping he or she would think she was a co-worker; the upturned jacket collar covered the lower half of her face, and the jacket was long enough to cover her thighs. Her ploy appeared to work; the figure waved back, then returned to their cigarette.

Willing herself to stay calm and ignoring significant discomfort, Lussi walked as fast as she was able to her left, past the yellow loader, and around the side of the hangar. She sank into the jacket and, with her hands in her pockets, made for a parking lot she remembered was close to the far end of the hangar. She'd parked in that lot six months ago. Behind her, she heard the engine of the loader start up.

On the right, a high metal fence topped with coils of barbed wire separated her from East Key Highway and a double railway track. The highway terminated at the entrance to the parking lot and, as far as Lussi was aware, this was the only exit from the Domino's compound that did not entail crossing multiple rail lines. As she passed the far corner of the hangar she could see to her left, through a forest of cranes and derricks, the bridge of a cargo ship at the dock. She turned right toward the car park.

Crossing the car park at an unhurried pace, both to attract as little attention as possible and because it was painful to walk any faster, Lussi encountered no one on foot. The gates were open, and a stream of cars were entering.

She breathed a sigh of relief as she reached the gates and turned right onto East Key Highway. Some distance ahead was a sharp left-hand turn in the road, where the three rail tracks exiting the Domino compound joined the main rail track. From here, she thought it was approximately half a mile to Ann's home. Her estimated time of arrival would be cutting it close.

Rain began to drizzle from a darkening sky, enhancing the gloominess of Lussi's view of the sugar factory from outside the perimeter fence. Corroded vehicles and other metal objects were intermixed with modern truck and train containers and predominantly dilapidated buildings.

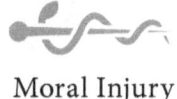

Approximately 8:15 a.m.

ANN CASTLE LIVED IN THE MIDDLE OF A BLOCK OF ROW houses. Her home stood out from the others as the only one with a brick exterior, rather than the ubiquitous, multicolored faux stone facing applied to eighty percent of the row houses in Baltimore. Lussi's heart sank when she saw a dry area on the road in front of Ann's house where a car had recently been parked.

Damn it. I've just missed her.

Just in case, Lussi climbed the worn marble steps to the front door and rang the doorbell; there was no response. She walked to the far end of the row and entered the back alley. There was no car parked beside Ann's diminutive backyard. Over her back door was a green and white striped metal awning; Lussi sank onto the steps beneath it. The kitchen, visible through a full-length reinforced glass door, was dark and empty.

The shelter from the awning proved purely psychological; Lussi's head and legs were wet and sticky, and there was enough solid raw sugar remaining in her underclothes to make sitting uncomfortable. It was difficult to focus on developing a backup plan when she felt so hungry, cold, and uncomfortable.

No one else I know lives in this area, and I can't stay here long.

It was impossible to miss the multiple signs heralding the *Neighborhood Watch*. Three people had already passed by in the alley and stared at Lussi questioningly.

Huddled with her back against the door, her forehead resting on her knees, Lussi was jolted from her misery by forceful thudding. Ann was banging with her knuckles on the inside of the kitchen door, threatening to call the police.

Lussi stood up, turned around, and pulled down her jacket collar. A look of astonishment replaced anger on Ann's face as she hurriedly unlocked the door.

"Oh my God Lussi! What's happened to you?" Ann caught Lussi in her arms as she almost fell through the door. The strength that had enabled Lussi to escape from the sugar factory had vanished.

After half dragging Lussi to a chair, Ann brought her a glass of water.

"We've been so worried about you."

Ann stroked Lussi's hands and her cheeks. "You're so cold. Don't talk now. Let's get you into a warm bath. I just came home to pick up the ferrets for the intubation workshop at South Baltimore. I'll call and cancel the workshop after I run you a bath."

Lussi spoke for the first time. The raw sugar had excoriated the inside of her throat and nose, so her voice was low and grating. "What day is this? How long have I been missing?"

"I don't know exactly. You told me you were going over yesterday to meet with the lab director at South Baltimore. I assumed that he would take you on a tour of the facility, and maybe have you meet colleagues, so I wasn't really expecting to see you in the afternoon. I *was* a little surprised when you didn't call to let me know how the meeting went, but I figured you were in a hurry to get home. Did something happen at South Baltimore?"

"Yes. I don't think you should cancel the workshop. I promise you I will be fine while you drop off the ferrets. Ask one of the other demonstrators to run the workshop. You can say you are not feeling well and need to go home. Just please don't mention that you've seen me. When you get back, I will tell you what happened. May I use your phone to call Howard and the kids?"

"You might not want to call just yet, Lussi, if you don't want people at South Baltimore to know you're here. Police are stationed at your house, and they'll report that you've been found."

"It is not only the people at Southern Baltimore, Ann; I'm pretty sure Children's Hospital personnel are also involved." Lussi folded herself into a fetal position in the large armchair.

Ann put on the kettle. "I'm going to make you a cup of sweet tea, which you will drink while I run your bath and find towels and clean clothes for you. The bed in the guest-room is already made up. I'll get the ferrets delivered and be back as quickly as I can. I'll find a way to contact your family without alerting the police. Don't worry."

Lussi nodded.

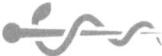

11:45 a.m.

Lussi was awoken by the doorbell. She could hear Howard talking to Ann downstairs.

Howard, who was approaching the bottom of the stairs as Lussi started to descend, came to an abrupt standstill when he saw her.

Lussi hesitated. "Don't be upset by how I look, Howard. All things considered; I was fortunate. I got knocked out and my shoulder is injured, but the other damage is only skin deep. What about Rachel and John; are they at home?"

"Yes. The police say they can't allow them to go to school until they get a better handle on your case. Ann called me at home and told the policewoman who answered the phone that she was *my* colleague and just wanted to check how I was holding up."

"I called him from an empty office in building C where we are holding the ferret workshop. Howard was very cool and accepted my call without question, so the policewoman left him alone to talk to me."

Howard added, "I haven't told the kids yet – I wanted to see and talk to you first Lussi. The police think I'm dealing with something urgent at work."

Howard and Ann listened in silence to Lussi's description of events, starting with her interview at Kader's laboratory and concluding at Ann's kitchen door.

"These people are obviously quite willing to kill to protect their secret," Howard observed. "As you said, Lussi, this has major implications for how we go about informing the police. We cannot let the perpetrators discover you are alive."

"Have the police told you whether they have any clue what might have happened to me?" Lussi asked.

"No, but judging from the questions they asked me, they are thinking there might be a link to the kidnapping from the Children's car park or to my work at Fort Dietrick. They are screening all calls and believe there will be a ransom call."

"Ransom? Is that what they think is behind this?" Lussi could hear her voice rising. "Why are the police wasting time on that theory? We are far from millionaires. Oliver Turner was stolen from his parents, and they think he's *dead*. We've got to get moving and rescue those babies from South Baltimore Hospital."

Ann and Howard exchanged glances; Howard said gently, "Well, it's not as if the police know anything about what's going on at South Baltimore, Lussi, and, although I revealed to them the minimum detail about my work at Fort Dietrick, I did tell them it was hush-hush and of potential interest to unfriendly foreign entities."

Lussi nodded wearily. "I know, I've no reason to rail at the police and I apologize for unloading on you guys. But I *must* report the whole story as soon as possible. Can we drive to the police station now?"

Ann said, "It's already evening, and you've only slept for a couple of hours Lussi. You can't go home tonight, with the house under surveillance, so stay here and get some rest."

Howard nodded. "That's an excellent plan Lussi. You should talk to *senior* police officers, who are less likely to be physically present at the station overnight, and there will be personnel immediately available in the morning who have the ability to develop a rescue plan that does not further endanger either you or the infants at South Baltimore. I'll pick you up and take you to the police station early tomorrow morning."

Chapter 14

Wednesday, February 25th, 1987, 6:30 a.m.

BILL SCHULTZ ROLLED OUT OF BED, RELEASING A WAVE of relief across the overburdened mattress, and waking his wife, Donna. Donna, with expertise gained from frequent practice, pretended to be asleep. Bill pressed a switch at his side of the bed and Donna heard the TV console rising from the bedroom floor at the foot of the bed.

Just like a coffin ascending from the inferno – hideous thing.

Bill turned on his favorite news program and proceeded to complete his morning ablutions with the bathroom door open, making no attempt to dampen the accompanying acoustics.

It had been several years since Donna had felt the need to prepare breakfast for Bill.

His ultra-high-tech automatic coffee maker, along with his daily morning delivery of fresh croissants, does a far better job of satisfying his needs than I ever have.

Bill and she had been married for thirty-seven years. It had come as no surprise to Donna that, as Bill's financial portfolio grew, so did his magnetic attraction for female predators. She was fully aware that Bill had, on several occasions, planned to trade her in for a younger model, but his intentions had somehow never come to fruition.

He probably decided it wasn't worth the bother.

After all, she didn't spend his money – she had plenty

of her own – and she had no desire to be constantly in touch with his whereabouts. She was also aware that she possessed an intangible asset, *class,* and it never let him down at social events.

Bill was openly proud of his core personality traits, which he readily acknowledged included arrogance, avarice, cunning, callousness, and aggressiveness. He referred to those not possessing these attributes as "Schmucks."

I did love Bill in the beginning. Then, over time, I just learned to live with his narcissism. When I'm asked why I stay with him I say I love the freedom from responsibility to please, responsibility to share, and responsibility to understand. But if I'm honest, it's my way of getting revenge.

Donna was awoken again by the sound of the front door opening and closing downstairs. Bill was on his way to pick up Suzanne Sinclair for their commute to Children's Hospital.

It was a mystery to me why Bill, who loathes children, moved us here from Texas to head up a Children's Hospital. But I didn't know then that Suzanne was joining us. I feel so sorry for George. He's such a decent man and it would break his heart if he knew.

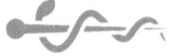

6:58 a.m.

SUZANNE WAS SITTING ON THE WALL OUTSIDE THE ELECtronic gate of her estate. On seeing Bill's car approaching she tossed her cigarette butt into a bush, then slid off the wall, in the process allowing her skirt to rise above her uncovered crotch. She neglected to pull down her skirt prior to bending over to pick up her briefcase and purse.

Suzanne opened the passenger side door, climbed in, and sat down. Bill made no effort to control himself, lunging at Suzanne and then forcing his index finger under her skirt and into her vagina. She pulled Bill's hand away and demanded that he drive to their usual spot in the woods.

Following the sex, the commute evolved into a one-sided litany of complaints from Bill.

"It's been an abysmal week so far, Suzanne; the Sim woman's vanishing stunt, then police milling all over both hospitals demanding to interview everyone, down to the janitorial staff. On top of it all, Don Evans at South Baltimore is acting like he's losing it – hiding in his office and not doing his job. I feel like I'm his fucking psychiatrist. So, I've scheduled a meeting with him this morning and want you to be there."

"What time is your meeting, Bill? I've got a full schedule."

"Eight fifteen."

"I wish you'd told me earlier, Bill. I've got a budget review meeting with Surgery set up for that time. Why do you want me there anyway? I have nothing to do with the running of South Baltimore, and the only time I've met Don Evans was at the hospital opening celebration."

"Well Suzanne, *darling*, I've got a most important favor to ask."

Oh God. Bill never asks, he commands. And 'darling' – really? Bill usually prefers more sexually explicit terms of endearment. Perhaps he thinks his sexual prowess has induced such a fantastic afterglow that I'll agree to anything.

"You are the only person with the expertise and brain power to pull this off, Suzanne."

"OK." Suzanne paused. "Tell me what this favor is, and I will think about it."

"As I was telling you, this business with Lussi Sim is getting out of hand over at South Baltimore hospital, mainly because of that spineless idiot, Don Evans. He has no guts or street smarts. I need to distance myself from him and keep myself out of the limelight over there, for the sake of the reputation of Children's Hospital. I don't want the police to get the idea that any of us are involved in the disappearance of Dr. Sim. I need to back off a bit, and you are the perfect person to step in and help Don to pull things together. As you pointed out, you haven't been involved with the running of his hospital, even in an advisory role, so you are 'clean' as far as the police are concerned."

"I don't relish walking blindly into the middle of a police investigation, Bill. How am I going to assist when I have no idea what is going on?" She emphasized the last point as though she thought he was intentionally keeping her in the dark.

"Suzanne, I've no idea why the police are leaning on Don so hard, but I do know that he is a hell of a lot more likely to make things worse than better. You have knowledge and experience that will enable him to deal with the police without revealing to them what a dribbling moron he is."

Suzanne was not reassured. "I need time to think this over, Bill, it seems to me I could end up as a scapegoat for something I know nothing about."

"Jesus, Suzanne, there's no fucking chance of that. When the police question me tomorrow, I'll make it clear that this is a temporary role for you; you've never been an employee of South Baltimore Community Hospital and are simply on loan to help Don respond to their requests. I need your answer before we reach the hospital. We are meeting with Don at eight-fifteen."

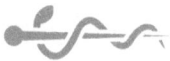

8:10 a.m.

DON EVANS WAS VISIBLY AGITATED WHEN HE ARRIVED for the meeting. His face and jowls were coated with a patina of sweat, his silk suit was wrinkled, and the ends of his tie dangled from a jacket pocket. Remarkably, Suzanne thought, considering the hour, Bill offered Don a whiskey, which he accepted. Bill did not fix himself a drink or offer one to her, but he poured a double for Don.

"Of course," Bill started right in, "I don't need to remind you, Don, that 'loose lips sink ships.' Following our conversation yesterday, I have asked Suzanne to assist you with the practicalities of relating to the police in a proficient manner. Kader will help you deal with any international stuff. Your customary lack of take-charge behavior will merely serve to convince the police that you are a viable suspect in the disappearance of Dr. Sim. Also, in the meanwhile, the less we appear to be in each other's pockets the better.

"Thankfully, you were able to get the Sim woman's car out of the parking lot before the police arrived. With her car gone, there's no indication that she was even at South Baltimore when she disappeared. The police seem to be basing their investigation on the theory that her disappearance is linked to the abduction from our parking garage at Children's. Let's keep it that way."

Suzanne had, up to this point, been listening stone-faced.

Well now, this is interesting. What are these guys trying to cover up? This isn't just about Lussi Sim; Bill appears to be into something with Don that I've failed to uncover. Something he is anxious to hide from the police. Perhaps this assignment will turn out to be more productive than I thought.*

She smiled at Don and said, "I am happy to help, Don, and, of course, you will remain fully in charge of things at South Baltimore."

Don did not return her smile. Responding with slumped shoulders and an air of resignation, he said, "Thank you, Ms. Sinclair, for taking time out of your busy schedule. I agree with Bill that he and I should keep some distance between us for a while. I haven't any experience dealing with a police investigation, so your assistance will be most welcome."

Suzanne struggled with an urge to laugh.

Don had an erection and his hands all over me when I met him at the South Baltimore Hospital opening celebration. A few days later, Bill told me that Don remarked to him that, while I am "easy on the eyes," I am categorically an "Ice Maiden."

"Well, since we are all in agreement, I'll leave you and Ms. Sinclair to work out the details, Don."

"Please hang on a minute, Bill." Don almost wiped his brow with his tie. "The police have informed me that Dr. Sim told members of her staff that she was going to meet with Paul Kader at his laboratory on the day she disappeared. Kader has confirmed that she had an appointment but says she never turned up. This was verified by Kader's secretary. However, one of our NICU nurses told the police she'd directed Dr. Sim to Building C, next door to the research laboratories, just a few days before she disappeared. Now the police are asking me questions I can't answer about Building C.

"When you offered me the CEO position, you led me to believe that Building C contained conference rooms and some undesignated 'reserve space' for use as the hospital grew. I showed the police the plans you gave me, but they seem to think I'm hiding something. Is there something going on in that building that I and Ms. Sinclair should know about?"

It was obvious to Suzanne that Bill choked back a retort, before responding in an uncharacteristically measured tone. "Now Don, let's back up a bit. You are quite happy to share in the financial largess of our foreign investors, no questions asked. The eventual utilization of the reserve space in Building C, as I told you when you took the job as CEO, is a clinical decision. You are not a clinician. However, if you had asked for details, I'd have been happy to provide them. It is my clear recollection that you did not ask, and there is nothing further that you need to know at this juncture."

Don stared at Bill with his mouth open.

"As it turns out Don, it seems to me that the less you know the better. You won't have to lie. I strongly suggest you do as I say and cooperate fully with Ms. Sinclair. She has expertise in dealing with the authorities, including the police. Her lack of involvement with the running of South Baltimore can only serve to enhance your claimed lack of involvement in Dr. Sim's disappearance."

"I'll try my best."

"Believe me, Don. You had better do a great deal more than *try*." Bill leaned forward to turn on one of his two desk-top computers, which commenced to boot up noisily, making further conversation difficult.

The executive floor was the only area in the hospital equipped with computers. Suzanne was aware that Bill had demanded that the Children's Hospital board of trustees provide him with a Macintosh computer with connectivity to the nascent internet, while hers and the other executive offices were on an IBM intranet system which Bill could access from his second terminal.

With his eyes fixed pointedly on the screen Bill was obviously declaring the meeting adjourned. Don crept out of the office, closing the door softly behind him. Bill rocked back in his chair, placed his fingertips together, flexed and extended his fingers pensively, and turned to Suzanne.

"Don cannot resist whining at every opportunity. Deal with him firmly, Suzanne. He's a loose cannon and I can't take his bleating much longer. When this mess is over, he is history."

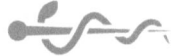

9:00 a.m.

HOWARD, LUSSI, AND ANN CASTLE TOOK THEIR SEATS around a table in the office of Colonel Sylvia Parker, Baltimore Metropolitan Police.

Lussi thought Colonel Parker could best be described as "regal". A tall, slim African American woman, with distinguished bearing, wearing a police uniform displaying abundant gold braid around her cuffs and on her cap. Also at the table, but not in uniform, was a white male whom the colonel introduced as Detective Lieutenant Strand.

Having listened in silence to their story, Colonel Parker removed her glasses and rubbed her eyes.

"Frankly, what you've told me sounds bizarre, however, I'm inclined to believe you. I can't figure out what any of you would gain from making this up."

Glancing over at Lieutenant Strand, the colonel asked, "Do you agree with me, Lieutenant, that, while acknowledging the urgency of this situation, if we rush in too fast, we run the risk of, at the very least, causing additional injury to the patients in this unit?"

"Absolutely Colonel, this intervention will require meticulous planning, in close cooperation with the SWAT team, and qualified medical and nursing personnel."

The colonel turned to Lussi. "Dr. Sim, it does appear that the perpetrators both wanted you dead and believe you are dead. Thus, revealing that you're alive will simply alert them to cover their tracks and may put you at risk once again."

"I'm afraid so, Colonel," Lussi replied. "I agree with you and Lieutenant Strand; we need to plan together to optimally protect the patients. NICU staff from Children's will have to be standing by at South Baltimore to take care of the infants in the unit after it is secured."

"I will rely on your expert advice when we reach that stage, Dr. Sim, but allow us to complete our preliminary plans for the police operation before additional personnel are involved. We can't afford to do anything that might alert the perpetrators. Of course, Ms. Castle may keep her ears and eyes open at work but please, nothing more. While I was listening to your story, I made a list of those who struck me as possible suspects."

Colonel Parker went over to a copier and made four copies of a single sheet. "You'll see that I've divided my list based on whether the potential suspect is an employee of Children's or South Baltimore Hospital; you have convinced me that personnel from both institutions are probably involved.

Under Children's Hospital, I've listed Bill Schultz, CEO, Suzanne Sinclair, CFO, Dr. Azad Sula, Neonatologist, and Dr. Christian Carter, Pediatric Heart Surgeon. Under

South Baltimore General Hospital are, Don Evans, CEO, Dr. Naeem Daher, Neonatologist, and Dr. Paul Kader, Research Laboratory Director. Of course, there are likely to be additions, and this list is intended as a guide to those who should be placed under continuous surveillance immediately. Do any of you feel that I should add anyone else? Dr. Sim; go ahead."

"I would add Tony Blake, the COO at Children's Hospital. He is Bill Schultz's hatchet man. What about you, Ann? Should she add any of the nursing staff?"

Ann said, "I would add Dr. Sally Wright, Cardiologist at Children's; her behavior was so strange the night I picked up Baby Turner. It is going to be important to keep the Children's Hospital Director of Nursing, Sherry Dunstan, from knowing that we are recruiting nurses and other staff to deal with the transfer of patients from South Baltimore to Children's, mostly because she can be counted on to alert Bill Schultz. However, although she worships Bill and parrots what he tells her to, I can't imagine him buddying up with her as a co-conspirator."

"I agree with Ann about both Sally Wright and Sherry Dunstan, Colonel." Said Lussi.

Colonel Parker pushed back her chair. "Thank you all for your input. Please keep my office informed of any developments that might impact our planning, which will commence immediately. You have indicated that for the time being, Dr. Sim will be staying at Ms. Castle's home and have provided contact information – in turn, we have provided you with direct and emergency contact information for both of us. Dr. Sim and Ms. Castle, would you please draft a plan for the transfer of the infants from the South Baltimore unit to Children's

Hospital and get it to me as soon as possible, along with the key to Building C."

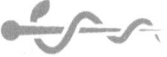

6.15 p.m.

Colonel Parker had emphasized the importance of taking no action that might alert the perpetrators. While Lussi had every intention of adhering to this instruction, she realized that the possession of the key to Building C and the fact that Ann had legitimate access could be of immediate value to them. To hand over a key to the police was certainly a pending imperative. However, at this early stage of planning it did not seem wise to have a police officer enter Building C and risk discovery. Ann immediately concurred with Lussi's line of reasoning and drove to Building C ostensibly to feed and water the ferrets.

Meanwhile, under the pretext of escorting them to an after-school event, Howard brought John and Rachel over to Ann's home for a short, but jubilant, reunion with their mother. Howard reported that he had overheard the two police officers stationed at their house discussing Lussi's car. Her vehicle had been discovered out in Sparrow's Point by a security guard at the Bethlehem Steel factory, on the construction site for a new blast furnace.

By the time Ann arrived home from building C at seven twenty-five p.m., Lussi was apprehensive, while Ann was highly energized and eager to report her findings.

"Just as we discussed, Lussi, I hid in the kitchen across the corridor from the restricted access door. With the kitchen door open just a crack I could observe both the door opposite me and the keypad. I must say, as time passed it felt more and more like an incredible long shot, but at about six-thirty-five two men in white coats arrived at the door and used the keypad. They had their backs to me, but I could clearly see the numbers they punched in."

"Then Plan A is 'on' for tonight, Ann. Great work."

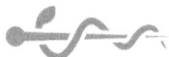

7.45 p.m.

Suzanne Sinclair was in a small, windowless, locked room inside the Sinclair stables. It had been easy for Suzanne to appropriate this space for her personal use without George being aware. He rarely visited the stables.

Lined with deep shelves on three sides and lit by a single light bulb, the small room smelt pleasantly of cedar. In addition to the worn leather armchair in which she was seated, other contents of the room included scattered books and manuals on wall shelves and a telephone and scrambler on a circular wooden table. Also on the table were three thick manuals, several well-sharpened pencils, an open spiral-bound notebook, an ashtray, a cigarette lighter, a full shot glass, a half-empty bottle of whiskey, and a short-wave radio.

Suzanne picked up the telephone and placed it in the scrambler cradle, before dialing and reading from her handwritten notes on a page torn from the spiral notebook. "Uncle seriously unwell. Unaware of precise diagnosis. Participants include Southern entities. The number/identity of other participants is unknown. Request direction."

Mhairi Haarsager, M.D.

Suzanne hung up the phone and took a sip of the whiskey in the shot glass, before tearing up the page from the notebook, crushing it, placing it in the ashtray, and using the lighter to set it alight.

Several minutes later the short-wave radio crackled. Suzanne grabbed a pencil and the notebook and wrote down the numbers provided, in sets of five, in a monotonous voice competing with copious white noise. Having reviewed these numbers, she tore the page from the notebook and disposed of it as before.

Chapter 15

Thursday, February 26th, 1987, 2:00 a.m.

From the kitchen in Building C, Lussi, and Ann, dressed in scrubs, head covers and masks watched the double metal doors across the corridor for fifteen minutes. No one left or entered. Ann punched the code into the keypad. The doors opened into a short, carpeted corridor leading to the center of an oblong lobby. To their left was an elevator; to their right a door labeled, SURGERY VIEWING ROOM.

Entering the viewing room, they found themselves in a semi-circular auditorium with four rows of benches descending on each side, separated in the center by steps heading down to a floor-to-ceiling, concave observation window that filled the entire front wall and emitted a dull glow. The window provided an expansive view of a dimly lit operating theater below, with two operating tables set up, each with an anesthesia machine at its head. In addition to multiple intravenous poles and monitors, there were two bypass pumps for heart surgery.

From the curved windowsill, Lussi picked up a clipboard holding a single sheet of paper. Sinking onto a front bench, she gestured to Ann to join her. The list was organized under five headings:

Date	Start Time	Donor	Recipient	Surgeon
2/18	6 a.m.	Infant AL	Infant MY	Christian Carter, M.D.*
3/02	6 a.m.	Infant OT	Infant M bin S	Christian Carter, M.D.*

*Assistant TBA

The second surgery was scheduled for just over three days from now, and the donor infant, OT, could only be Oliver Turner.

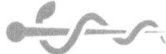

9:30 a.m.

FOR OVER AN HOUR AND A HALF, LUSSI AND ANN HAD been closeted with Colonel Parker in her office. Now the Colonel was presenting a summary of planning, to date, for *Operation Broken Hearts*, as she had formally designated it, based on the latest information from Ann and Lussi.

Colonel Parker initially reacted with anger to the early morning call from Lussi reporting what the Colonel made clear she considered a dangerous, rogue operation undertaken by two irresponsible, unqualified persons. Fortunately, she had cooled down considerably since then. With her now, seated around the conference table in her office, were Lieutenant Strand, Steve Cole, the director of the Special Weapons and Tactics (SWAT) team, Lussi, and Ann.

"Using building plans for the South Baltimore Community Hospital Campus obtained from City Hall, of which I have provided copies, Lieutenant Strand and I have been working with SWAT," Colonel Parker glanced at Steve Cole and smiled, "on how to gain undercover access to Building C and the research laboratories. Details of the insides of the buildings are missing from the plans, which are overall misleading. Building C is labeled *Future Expansion* and the inside is presented as empty space, and the research building is represented as having a single floor. We now know that it has at least three.

"While we have Dr. Sim and Ms. Castle to thank for providing information missing from the plans, I have emphasized to them that I shall have absolutely no tolerance for any further excursions like the one they made last night. They not only put themselves in danger but would have destroyed our chances to catch the perpetrators in the act, had they been discovered."

Lussi stared at the surface of the conference table, feeling like a schoolgirl being chastised by the headmistress. A warm smile from Steve Cole greeted her when she lifted her head.

This having been said," the Colonel continued, "the information provided by Dr. Sim and Ms. Castle is vital to the completion of a successful rescue plan. Our preliminary strategy is based largely upon their description of the layout of the inside of the two buildings, including what we now believe is a heart transplant unit. We have also obtained advice from experts on building design and construction. However, we require greater detail on the inside of the transplant unit to move the SWAT team safely into key positions without alerting the perpetrators.

"Now that we are in possession of a key to Building C, we can gain significant additional information from the measurement of the spaces separating doors, elevators, heating ducts, windows, stairways, etc., without leaving behind evidence of a break-in. Having the code for the keypad allows for a much higher level of planning precision."

"How long do you think it will take to complete your plan, taking into consideration what we now know about the timing of the next scheduled surgery?" Lussi asked, still feeling sheepish.

"I'll address this issue if I may, Colonel," said Steve Cole. "I know that completing our plan sounds like a lengthy, complicated procedure, doctor, but with the information you and Ms. Castle have provided, we should have the additional data we require in less than twenty-four hours. We intend to have the team members strategically placed inside the research building and Building C at least three hours prior to the start of surgery on Monday morning. Colonel Parker informs me that you two have outlined a preliminary plan for your side of the action. May we review that together now?"

He's both smart and personable. Lussi was heartened. "Yes, that would be fine. It is very much a first draft and, thus, includes a sizeable list of questions to be answered."

Colonel Parker distributed copies and asked Lussi to present the contents.

"There will be two five-member clinical teams. One, headed by Dr. Sim, will be responsible for rescue activities in the transplant operating room. The other, headed by Ann Castle, will be responsible for rescue activities in the transplant NICU.

"At an agreed time prior to the raid, four ambulances will be stationed close to, but outside, the perimeter of the South Baltimore Hospital campus. The ambulances will carry four transport nurses, two respiratory therapists, two neonatology fellows, Dr. Sim, Ms. Castle, and infant transport equipment. We will also carry the required sterile equipment. Because travel in this city can be significantly impeded by the volume of traffic during the morning rush hour, which begins early, a helicopter will be on standby at Children's Hospital in case more rapid transport is required for clinically unstable infants. There is a helicopter pad on the roof of South Baltimore Hospital.

"Neonatologist Mary Morrison, M.D., and Nurse Director of the NICU, Muriel Dressing will be responsible for the preparation of the NICU at Children's Hospital to receive the rescued infants. The NICU will be placed on *Bypass* status for patient referrals, to ensure that the NICU staff are able to admit and stabilize all the rescued infants before they resume accepting patients referred from other hospitals.

"You will see that under the heading 'Major Points for Discussion' we have listed five questions:

Question 1. Optimal number of members of the clinical rescue planning team?

The key underlying principle – keep numbers to the minimum possible: Mary Morrison, M.D. Neonatologist, Muriel Dressing, RN, Nursing Director of NICU, and a senior infection control nurse, as advisors. Ann Castle will select the four transport nurses and the respiratory therapists. So that their absence will not be missed, Lussi Sim will select two fellows who are not currently on duty in her NICU. Thus, ten healthcare personnel will ride in the ambulances, including herself and Ann.

"To avoid alerting an unknown perpetrator, we will not involve medical specialists from other services at Children's Hospital, such as surgery and cardiology, until the rescue operation is complete, and all the infants have been admitted to the Children's Hospital NICU."

Question 2. The optimal site, and the schedule for placement of the ambulances while waiting at South Baltimore?

Question 3.

A. Communication between the SWAT and the clinical teams before/during the raid?

B. Communication between clinical team leaders and Children's Hospital Transport Dispatch Center. Because the Children's NICU receives one hundred percent of patients as referrals from other hospitals, we have a highly sophisticated patient transport system in place. Ann and I will carry the cellular phones that are designated for use during patient transport. Will we need additional phones to contact SWAT, Steve?

Question 4. When and by what route/s will the clinical teams enter/leave the transplant unit?

A. From/to assigned ambulance.

B. To helicopter pad.

Question 5. Maintenance of Infection Control inside the transplant unit.

Ann and I will develop a plan with our senior Infection Control Nurse. We don't think it is necessary to supply you with the entire, detailed plan, which is much more likely to confuse than clarify. What we will do instead is prepare a list of precautions for the SWAT team so that they may avoid inadvertently breaking infection control protocol. Please contact me with any questions."

"Nice job emphasizing the essentials from the medical perspective," said Colonel Parker. "I have complete faith in both of you to select only those who are essential to the undertaking and whom you have known and worked with for long enough to gauge their trustworthiness. I assume the ambulances will be equipped with standard advanced life-support EMS radio equipment. The answers to questions two, three, and four require further thought and discussion on our side. Steve, may I refer Dr. Sim's question regarding communication with SWAT to you?"

"Absolutely Colonel. I am impressed by how much work has been accomplished on the plan in a short time, Dr. Sim. I commend the priority given to communication. Problems with rescue missions can more often be blamed on a failure in communication than any other component. I need to do a little homework on your question about phone communication with our team while you and Ms. Castle are inside the transplant unit. Would you supply me with contact information for your dispatch center?"

"I have a card in my purse which I carry with me at all times." Ann extracted the card and gave it to Steve. "Would you mind xeroxing it? I don't like to be without it."

"May I call you at four p.m. today, Dr. Sim?"

"Absolutely, colonel. I will be at Ann's home, so please use her phone number."

Chapter 16

Monday, March 2nd, 1987, 3:30 a.m.

LUSSI WAS TRAVELING IN THE LEAD AMBULANCE AS THEY silently departed Children's Hospital, their departure times staggered by the dispatcher with a three-minute gap. All four ambulances were equipped for advanced infant life support and carried EMS communications pre-programmable radios, set to EMS, UHF, VHF bands, and the specific bands utilized by SWAT. Lussi was carrying the cellular phone for her team – Ann for the other team.

These ambulances would wait in the designated location at the edge of the South Baltimore Hospital campus until Lussi received a call from Steve Cole indicating that they should move in. This phase of the raid had been thoroughly rehearsed.

Lussi was aware that, by two a.m. that morning, nine members of the SWAT team were in place on the roof of Building C, where, with cutting torches, they breached the metal door of the service entrance. Other members of the SWAT team entered the Research Building from Building C, using the keypad code. Once inside, the officers stationed themselves in the Surgical Viewing Room and in the ceiling of the corridors in the transplant unit, which Lussi recalled were finished with drop-in panels.

Additional police officers were hidden in Building C, outside the entrance to the research laboratories, immediately inside the entrance, and in the ladies' and men's rooms. The plan was to wait until most of the key personnel arrived, unless the transfer of Oliver Turner and the heart recipient from the NICU to the operating room was attempted earlier than expected. Lussi had instructed Steve Cole and Colonel Parker that the pump technicians would probably arrive about an hour and a half prior to the surgery, the operating room staff, anesthesiologist/s, assisting surgeon/s, and Dr. Christian Carter at least forty-five minutes prior to surgery.

At five fifteen a.m., Lussi received the awaited call. Staff pushing two occupied transport incubators had just come into view in the corridor between the NICU and the operating room. The SWAT team would deploy from the ceilings as soon as the infants were inside the operating room. At Lussi's signal, without lights or sirens, her ambulance passed through the rear hospital entrance reserved for trucks servicing the loading dock. The other ambulances followed.

Lussi's team entered via Building C and headed for the operating room; Ann's team entered through the Research Building and went to the NICU. In both cases, their passage was cleared for them by the police, who had doors open and elevators held.

It was clear that the SWAT officers had met with armed resistance. The bodies of two males dressed in scrubs, one of them still grasping a handgun, sat hunched against the left-hand wall of the corridor – heads drooping onto their chests. A second weapon lay amongst the widely scattered wedges of fractured mineral fiber ceiling tile that crunched underfoot. Incongruously, Lussi felt a stab of guilt as she passed the bodies, but she did not slow down.

The scene when Lussi and her team entered the operating room was surreal. A SWAT officer, wearing a surgical mask, head and shoe covers, and scrubs, identified herself and her partner. She had her weapon trained on several individuals lying face down on the floor. Her partner, a similarly attired male officer, was holding a handgun on three hospital staff who remained standing. Two of the three appeared to be the nurses attending to the two motionless infants on ventilators lying on the operating tables under heat lamps.

The male officer addressed Lussi.

"Doctor, I have made it clear to these three individuals that they *will* cooperate with you to prepare these patients for transfer out of here. As you requested, two are OR nurses and the third is an anesthesiologist. According to the anesthesiologist, the patients are receiving standard sedation for ventilator care; neither has yet received anesthesia for surgery. The surgeon, Christian Carter was arrested in the NICU, the assistant surgeon made an armed attempt to resist arrest. You will have passed his body in the corridor. There are police colleagues ready to help us take all these individuals into custody, however, to abide by your infection control guidelines, the two of us will maintain the status quo in here until you are ready to leave with the patients."

Lussi could see that Oliver Turner was on the table to her left and the infant who was to have received Oliver's heart, to her right. The latter infant was blue around the lips, with one of his three monitors sounding an intermittent alarm. Lussi and her transport nurse headed over to the heart recipient, while her fellow and the second transport nurse took care of Oliver.

Lussi addressed the anesthesiologist. "Doctor, please write me a list of the current intravenous medications, the dose each infant is receiving, and the time that the most recent dose was administered."

The male SWAT officer indicated with a small, but effective, motion of his firearm that this request must be responded to immediately and the anesthesiologist proceeded to comply.

The transport nurse was attempting to extract current clinical information from the distraught and frightened OR nurse caring for the recipient infant. This attempt was evidently unsuccessful since she quickly resorted to reading the nursing records attached to a clipboard lying on the operating table near the patient. In a corner of the OR, Lussi was relieved to see patient record files and X-ray packets lying on top of the transport incubators that delivered the infants to the OR.

Predictably, because of his relatively stable clinical condition, Oliver Turner was ready to leave before Lussi's patient. Lussi instructed the fellow to retrieve Oliver's X-rays from the viewing board and, with his transport nurse, move him to their assigned ambulance and leave immediately for Children's Hospital. The ambulance driver would inform the hospital transport dispatcher that they were on the way.

Lussi and her transport nurse worked on their patient for approximately fifteen additional minutes before Lussi felt that the patient was sufficiently stable to be moved. She called the dispatcher to send the waiting helicopter over from Children's and indicated to the SWAT officers that they were ready to leave. Replacing the X-rays and patient record on top of the transport incubator, Lussi and the nurse moved their patient out of the OR.

The two hunched bodies in the corridor had not changed position, but the pools of blood on the floor around them had expanded.

The transport nurse was handling the front end of the incubator, Lussi the rear. As they approached the far end of the corridor, from somewhere behind Lussi there was the muffled sound of a shot, followed by the OR door slamming shut. She and the nurse were now running with the incubator – Lussi pushing the incubator with one hand on the patient's file and X-rays to prevent them from falling and the nurse pulling the incubator with one hand and the IV pole with the other.

Suddenly, Lussi was grabbed by the shoulders from behind, pulled away from the incubator, and thrown against the corridor wall. Her scream brought the transport nurse to a halt.

Clutching the patient file, which she had somehow managed to hold onto as the packet of X-rays fell to the floor, Lussi hit the wall hard but did not lose consciousness. She slid her back against the wall, holding the file against her chest with both arms, until she was standing, propped against the wall, facing her attacker. He was wearing scrubs and a surgical mask and had a gun with a silencer pointed at her head.

"Do not move, keep your hands visible and I will not hurt you. Tell your nurse to stay where she is, or I will shoot her." Lussi recognized his voice and slight accent – it was the anesthesiologist.

She called to the nurse, keeping her voice as steady as she could. "Cathy, hold up a minute while I sort this out."

The anesthesiologist was now waving his gun at the nurse. "She will bring the child back here to me. *Tell her – NOW.*"

"The baby is critically unstable. If you delay our departure any longer, he will die. Is that what you want?" Lussi asked calmly.

Her apparent calm seemed only to engender increased agitation in the anesthesiologist. "My prince *will* have a new heart, or I will die for him in the name of Allah, and you will die with me."

The pounding of running feet could now be heard drawing nearer, from somewhere ahead of the transport nurse.

With her arms extended in front of her, holding the bulky patient record file in both hands, Lussi spun her body fast and let go of the file, shouting, "Run, Cathy!" The file hit the anesthesiologist square on his chest causing him to drop the gun, which landed some distance away. Lussi lunged to retrieve the weapon just as a SWAT officer grabbed the anesthesiologist and threw him face down on the floor. Seconds later, two EMS personnel squeezed past them pushing a gurney loaded with equipment toward the OR.

Later that day Lussi was informed by Colonel Parker that, after she left the OR, the anesthesiologist overpowered the male SWAT officer and took his gun. The female officer aimed her weapon at the anesthesiologist, who shot her in the abdomen. She was currently in critical condition, undergoing surgery at Johns Hopkins Hospital. Fortunately, the male officer was able to retrieve her gun and maintain order in the OR until help arrived.

In addition to this episode, there had been earlier resistance from two, armed healthcare workers outside the OR. Both men had been shot and killed. One of them was believed to be the surgeon scheduled to assist Christian Carter with the heart transplant.

Three men attempted to escape via the ladies' restroom but were apprehended by police as they tried to leave the research building. An officer was slashed with a scalpel during their arrest.

By seven a.m., all four infants in the transplant unit had been transported safely to Children's Hospital, three by road ambulance under police escort, and one by helicopter.

By nine a.m., Lussi and the Children's Hospital Chaplain were at the Turner home. Although Oliver's parents were expecting them, they had not been told the reason for the visit.

Mr. Turner met them at the door in a dressing gown and pajamas, his face so pale and drawn that Lussi almost didn't recognize him.

"Please forgive me for greeting you in my night clothes. My wife is unwell. I help her to get up in the morning and make breakfast for her, then her sister comes over. My employer has been so kind and allows me to arrive late."

"Don't worry, Mr. Turner, we understand." Mr. Turner's worn appearance had given Lussi an idea. "I think it might be a good idea if I have a short chat with you in private before I explain why we are here to your wife. Will that be OK with you? You have both met our hospital Chaplain before – I thought she could say hello to Mrs. Turner while we talked. She does know we're coming?"

Mr. Turner put his hand against the door frame for support. "Yes, yes, doctor, she does."

Straightening up, he pointed to the kitchen. "We can talk in there. My wife is in the living room to your right and her sister is with her."

As soon as he had closed the kitchen door behind them, Mr. Turner asked, "Is this more bad news, doctor? If it is, please just tell me – I don't think it is a good idea to tell my wife – she is very depressed."

"It is good news, but it *will* come as a shock. That is why I suggested we talk first. Shall we sit down?"

Lussi quickly summarized the events leading to the discovery that Oliver was alive and his rescue, and told his father he was doing well at Children's Hospital.

Lussi thought that Mr. Turner took her news amazingly well. He was initially lost for words, but then he grabbed her hand and shook it vigorously.

"Although you must be bursting with questions, I don't want to leave your wife in suspense longer than necessary. I wonder, if we join her in the living room now, Mr. Turner, before we explain would you tell your wife that our news will make her happy?"

Now smiling broadly, Mr. Turner stood and headed for the kitchen door.

Chapter 17

Monday, March 2nd, 1987, 6:55 a.m.

The phone rang as Suzanne was putting on her coat.

Bill offered no greeting, instead launching directly into a proclamation. "Suzanne, I've decided to work from home today, so you should take the day off."

"But Bill, I don't have any of my files here and I've several meetings scheduled. I can drive myself to work. I've got to go to South Baltimore early anyway."

"Suzanne, this is not a request. You will remain at home or consider yourself fired." Bill hung up on her.

George was reading the morning paper in the kitchen as Suzanne crept out of the house and made for the stables. There was a stable-hand cleaning stalls at the other end of the building, but Suzanne had no trouble reaching her destination without being seen. She locked the door, sat down, and used the cradled phone. "Uncle highly disturbed. Recently uncovered plan not going well. Request urgent liaison with Max." Suzanne hung up the phone.

Fifteen minutes later, Suzanne was pulling out of her driveway. As she slowed the car to pass through the electric gate, she leaned over to the glove compartment to retrieve a handgun and a silencer.

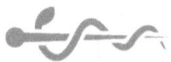

9:25 a.m.

Suzanne was in her office at Children's Hospital, wrapping up a meeting with Sherry Dunstan before driving to South Baltimore Hospital, when her phone buzzed. Don Evans was on the line – barely coherent. Suzanne held her hand over the receiver until Sherry had left the room, then managed to halt Don in mid-ramble and ask him to slow down. Now she was able to decipher from the jumble of words, that the police had cordoned off buildings at South Baltimore Hospital and the entire hospital was on lockdown. Don insisted he had no idea what was going on, despite letting it slip that the police had informed him in person of their plan to allow nobody into the hospital unless they had been summoned to a patient emergency.

Rather than feeling grateful that she was prevented from going to South Baltimore, Suzanne was frustrated. Something underhand was going on over there and it was essential she discover what it was as quickly as possible. She made Don promise to let her know immediately when the Hospital reopened.

As she ended the call with Don, there was a knock at her office door and Joe Meridian rushed in.

"Hi, Suzanne. Where is everybody? Have you any idea what is going on in the NICU?"

Joe's face was flushed, and he was obviously exceedingly concerned.

Suzanne regarded Joe with an expressionless face. "I'm not sure to what you are referring, Joe."

Joe took the seat recently vacated by Sherry.

"At around seven fifteen a.m. today, I was called in from home by the on-call NICU fellow to examine four infants admitted to the NICU overnight from South Baltimore Community Hospital. Your office manager just informed me that Bill is out of the office all day, but you are covering for him. In case you were not aware, I am supposed to be notified in advance about all potential admissions from South Baltimore. I was not contacted prior to these transfers."

"Well, Joe, it's possible that the admissions have something to do with some sort of police action going on over at South Baltimore. Don Evans just called me about it but, to tell you the truth, he was not making a lot of sense. If I were you, I'd talk to Mary Morrison; she's covering for Lussi Sim. I'm sorry I can't be of further assistance – I must prepare for my ten o'clock appointment."

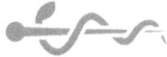

10:45 a.m.

At the Schultz residence the atmosphere could be cut with a knife. Donna had never seen Bill so agitated. Her attempts to communicate with him met with angry dismissal couched in vulgar language.

Bill hadn't left his home office in over three hours. When he finally came out and went to the kitchen, Donna made herself invisible. As he left the kitchen, carrying a can of soda, the phone in his office rang and, in his hurry to pick it up, Bill failed to completely close his office door behind him. Thus, Donna could clearly hear the ensuing conference call with Don Evans and Tony Blake.

"Goddammit Bill," Tony Blake started in on Bill without hesitation, "were you in on this transplant business?

Couldn't you have warned me? Rumors are running wild; they're saying that Christian Carter has been arrested."

"Hold it together, Tony," Bill ordered. "Don just joined the call. I did warn you not to go in to work today and there was no need for you to know about the transplant unit. We have limited time to plan our next move and to make sure that we get our stories straight. If we play our cards right, we can convince the police that rumors have suggested that financial backers approached Christian Carter after the shutdown of his heart transplant program at Children's, and none of us knows anything about the deal they made with him. Don, you will demonstrate to the police that the construction plans for Building C, supplied to you when you were appointed CEO, show the space as reserved for future expansion. Explain to them that you have never had a reason to visit what you understood was an empty building. Just as you have never found it pertinent to your job description to visit the research laboratories. Are we in agreement? How about you, Tony? Are you with us?"

"Since I am not a party to whatever scam you and Don are pulling at South Baltimore, Bill, I must respectfully decline your invitation. What the hell? Sounds to me like you guys are in deep trouble, of the sort that ends with long-term incarceration."

"Such righteousness, Tony, hardly becomes you. You damn well are involved – where did you think all those under-the-table bonuses came from? Certainly not from Children's Hospital profits. And you may rest assured that there is a clear paper trail attached to every payment, leading from the 'scam', as you call it, directly to your bank account."

Tony roared, "Fuck you – you bastard, you'll pay for this."

"I really don't think so, Tony. The people I'm working with

are experts at making people like you disappear, for good. I think, if you weigh the pros and cons carefully, you will conclude that remaining alive is the superior option. Now, back to you, Don. I don't recall hearing your answer to my question."

"Sure, Bill. I'm with you." Don's voice was a hoarse croak.

Bill continued. "Good to hear, Don. Just do exactly what I've told you to do."

"Have you lost your mind, Bill?" Tony bellowed. "I can't believe that you are relying on Don, that chicken shit asshole, to suddenly grow a spine and keep his cool under fire."

"Well Tony, it seems to me right now that Don's survival instinct is somewhat superior to yours. Are you with us or not?"

There was silence for what felt like an age to Donna but was probably measured in seconds.

"Won't it automatically arouse suspicion that both of us took today off." Tony stated rather than asking.

"I told my office manager that we needed peace and quiet to work together on an urgent project, Tony. Go back to work tomorrow. If you are asked about the project, we were working on the final phase of the Beltway Specialty Clinics scheme. Keep to this script and you will be fine."

By the time that Bill noticed his office door was ajar, Donna was weeding flower beds in the front garden, while trying to make sense of what she'd overheard.

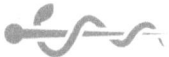

6:55 p.m.

DONNA WAS INCREASINGLY AWARE OF HER HUSBAND'S atypical behavior. This was far beyond Bill's usual level of self-absorbance and failure to communicate; there was superimposed anxiety and, she sensed, fear. This afternoon he'd spent hours in his office packing papers into boxes, which he then deposited in the trunk of his car. Now he was packing enough clothes for several days at least.

When Donna followed him outside to his car and asked where he was going, Bill bellowed at her. "For God's sake, woman leave me alone. The less you know, the better. I'll be back in a few days."

Charming as always. But this time whatever he is mixed up in sounds toxic. I've never seen him panic before.

Returning to the house, Donna watched Bill from the open front door.

Throwing the second of two suitcases into the trunk of his Mercedes, he closed it and walked toward the house with his raincoat over his arm. Reaching the driver's side door, Bill opened it and leaned in to toss his coat onto the passenger seat. Donna heard what sounded like a muffled shot that seemed to come from the rear of the house. Bill stood up slowly and closed the car door, shouting, "Goddamn hunters," and waving a fist toward the woods behind the house.

Bill pushed past Donna in the entrance hall and returned to his office, locking the door behind him. Donna assumed that he was making another telephone call. The grandfather clock in the entrance hall struck seven p.m. A minute later, Bill emerged from his office, relocked the door, and left the house without closing the front door.

Donna watched her husband reach for the driver's side door handle. Then something she couldn't identify caused him to turn toward the house with his right hand still on the door handle. He stared toward the rear of the house, a horrified glare frozen on his face. She heard again the muffled sound she'd heard earlier and then, to Donna it seemed in slow motion, a red circle appeared in the center of Bill's forehead and grew larger as he crumpled against the car door.

Ignoring the risk, Donna ran to Bill, felt his wrist for a pulse, and failed to find one. As she started to run back to the house to call 911, two men in dark suits with guns drawn ran after her.

One of the men shouted, "Police! Stay where you are." As they drew abreast of Donna, the second man said, "Mrs. Schultz, we've called emergency services and Ray here will do CPR until they arrive." The speaker continued to run toward the woods, while Ray holstered his weapon and ran over to Bill. Ray retrieved a small camera from a pocket, removed his jacket, and dropped it onto the driveway. After quickly taking two photographs of Bill from different angles, he placed him flat on his back, felt for a pulse in his neck, and began to perform chest compressions.

Donna stammered, "How did you get here so fast? I haven't had time to call for help."

"We were watching the house, ma'am," Ray said over his shoulder as he paused chest compressions to provide a mouth-to-mouth breath to Bill. "If you reach into the upper right pocket in my jacket, ma'am, you'll find my identification."

Donna retrieved the ID as instructed while the officer, identified as Detective Sergeant Raymond Cutler of the Baltimore police department, continued CPR.

The sound of sirens could be heard in the distance. Donna felt herself swaying sideways. For support, she grabbed the trunk of one of the trees lining the driveway.

Ray Cutler said, "Look, ma'am, you don't need to stay here. I've radioed Emergency Services and I'll do my best for your husband until they arrive. Why don't you go inside? I or my partner will come in and talk to you once the EMS team is here."

Donna nodded. As she turned to walk back to the house, the emergency vehicle arrived in the driveway behind her and she saw her neighbor, Suzanne Sinclair, hurrying toward her over the lawn. As Suzanne came closer, Donna could see that she was, as usual, dressed in expensive, fashionable clothes but she was barefoot, carrying a pair of stiletto-heeled shoes which she replaced on her feet before stepping from the lawn onto the driveway.

"I just heard the sirens and saw the ambulance pulling in here. Are you OK Donna?"

This is melodramatic. Donna unwound Suzanne from her torso. "I need to sit down."

Ray Cutler had now been relieved by two paramedics, who were applying electroshock to Bill's chest. Ray had his ID visible when he tapped Suzanne on the shoulder. "Excuse me, ma'am. Detective Sergeant Raymond Cutler, Baltimore Police. This is a crime scene. Please identify yourself and keep your hands visible."

Suzanne complied immediately. "I'm Suzanne Sinclair. My husband George Sinclair and I live next door." Suzanne pointed into the distance to the right of the Schultz residence.

"Well, Mrs. Sinclair, I would appreciate it if you would go into her house with Mrs. Schultz and find her something to drink. You will need to stay with her until my partner and I join you. We will also need to speak to your husband."

Suzanne put an arm around Donna's shoulders. "I'm happy to do that, officer. My husband left on a business trip this morning. I'm not sure when he will be back."

As Donna and Suzanne walked to the house, one of the paramedics came over to Ray Cutler, shaking his head. His partner had stopped doing CPR and was packing equipment.

Chapter 18

Tuesday, March 3rd, 1987, 2:10 p.m.

SITTING AT HER DESK, COLONEL SYLVIA PARKER CLASPED a mug of coffee to her chest with both hands and stared at the photographs spread out in front of her. Her eyes rested on an image of Bill Schultz slumped against his car. Bill's head drooped to the left, against the outside of the incompletely closed driver's-side door. Above him, a set of car keys dangled from the lock. Sylvia reviewed facts that were evident to date:

Fact-1: The bullet had entered Bill's forehead just above the bridge of his nose, exiting from the crown of his head. This bullet was recovered a few feet from his body, embedded in the trunk of a tree. According to forensics, this shot was fired from a high-powered rifle and, judging from the trajectory, in a semi-prone position.

On review of the ballistic evidence, the only additional information about the shooting, provided independently by Donna Schultz, Suzanne Sinclair, and the two responding police officers, was that the shot that killed Bill appeared to come from a densely wooded area behind the house. The meticulous search of the woods hadn't revealed any useful evidence. There were scattered hunter's hides and plentiful expended shells, but no spent cartridges that matched with the bullet that killed Bill Shultz. The only object that was possibly contemporaneous with the shooting and found in the area judged by forensics to be the site of origin of the bullet that killed Bill, was a children's toy – a tiny rubber lion bearing no retrievable fingerprints.

Fact-2: The police officers had not heard the first shot, reported by both Donna and Suzanne. At the time, they were changing shifts, and their cars were parked out on the main road.

Fact-3: Prior to his death, Bill Schultz was at home all day with his wife. Donna Shultz stated that it was most unusual for Bill to abruptly decide to take a day off work, although it was not out of character for him to plan a trip and not tell her where he was going. Approximately eight hours prior to the murder, Donna overheard her husband talking on the phone to 'Don' and 'Tony' about a transplant unit. She heard Tony threaten Bill, but Bill did not reveal any recognizable evidence over the phone that he was afraid of Tony. In fact, she thought he was in control of the conversation throughout. However, after that call, Donna said, her husband showed progressive signs of panic.

Why didn't Bill leave home earlier? If he was afraid of someone at Children's, possibly Tony Blake, although he has an apparently solid alibi, or wanted to avoid the police, why, when the location of his home is common knowledge among the medical and management staff, did he hang around for so long?

Fact-4: The papers found in Bill's car prove, without doubt, that he and Christian Carter were deeply involved in planning and running the covert transplant unit but, unfortunately, fall short of revealing the source of financing.

Fact-5: On the evening of Bill's death, Suzanne Sinclair arrived home at six fifty-three p.m. The first shot occurred at approximately six fifty-five. At seven p.m. the detectives who had followed Suzanne from Children's Hospital took over surveillance of both houses from the daytime crew.

Fact-6: The second shot was fired at approximately 7:03 p.m., following which detectives were at the crime scene in less than three minutes. Donna Schultz was the only eyewitness to the shooting. Cardiopulmonary resuscitation was attempted, but no pulse was ever detected despite repeated use of a cardiac defibrillator.

Fact-7: Suzanne Sinclair arrived at the scene of the shooting at approximately 7:08 p.m., at which time an ambulance was in the driveway, CPR was ongoing, and Donna Schultz was standing near her husband's body. Donna and Suzanne both tested negative for gunshot residue. Detective Sergeant Cutler and his partner reported that both women were cooperative and allowed them full access to their homes. Several appropriately registered firearms were retrieved from both houses; none had been recently fired.

When I interviewed Suzanne Sinclair on the evening of the shooting, I was struck by her intelligence and apparent desire to be helpful. She stated that, shortly after arriving home from work, she heard what sounded like a muffled shot coming from somewhere in the woods to the left of the rear of her house. She did not think much about it, because it was hunting season and she was accustomed to hearing shots fired in the woods. Although she also heard the second shot, she said she did not leave her house until she heard sirens. At the request of detective sergeant Ray Cutler, she accompanied Donna Schultz into her house and offered her a cup of tea, but Donna asked for whiskey.

Funny though, Suzanne described a genial, neighborly relationship with Donna but, although I can't pinpoint the specific language, I had the distinct impression that Donna *does not reciprocate Suzanne's cordial feelings.*

As it turns out, rather than release her on her own recognizance, I should have paid more attention to what Donna was implying and detained Suzanne for further questioning. Despite still being under surveillance, Suzanne did not appear for her second interview this morning and is now officially a missing person of interest. There are no indications that she has left Baltimore by air, road, water or rail.

Colonel Parker glanced at her watch.

I have an interrogation starting in fifteen minutes. I'd better get my thoughts centered on Chistian Carter and the transplant unit. Almost half the other staff arrested during the raid on the unit have undergone initial interrogation but, overall, things are not moving as fast as I would like.

The nursing staff and other non-physician healthcare providers, and the anesthesiologist arrested at the transplant unit, claim to know nothing about the evolution of the unit, which they state they believed to be a United States government-funded research institution. All these employees were interviewed for their positions at the same hotel in downtown Washington, DC, and they were all required to sign documents, ostensibly, but not in fact, issued by the National Institutes of Health, attesting to their understanding that this was a secret, top-priority research unit and that, by signing, they were agreeing to adhere to the listed requirements. Fulfillment of these requirements purportedly would lead to their being granted a mid-level government security clearance. Also listed were the formidable consequences of non-compliance, but the salary levels offered were so generous that it was, apparently, easy for the applicants to discount them.

Dr. Carter and the anesthesiologist independently admitted that they suspected the transplant unit was receiving funding from Saudi interests, but insisted they had never, personally, met with a representative of the Saudi Arabian government. In addition to the fact that the ethnicity of the anesthesiologist was obviously Semitic, and he had referred to the infant scheduled to receive Oliver Turner's heart as 'My Prince' and vowed to both die and kill for him in the name of Allah in Dr. Sim's presence, their statements were virtually identical and sounded rehearsed.

According to Carter, he was provided with signed parental consent for surgery for all the donor infants. Oddly, the only donor for whom any type of consent form could be found was Oliver Turner. However, this consent form was not for permission to allow Oliver to become a heart donor, but rather to enter him into a research project titled "Long-term Outcome of Male Versus Female Infants on ECMO."

Oliver's parents told police that they were asked to sign this form by one of the physicians, but they couldn't remember which one, shortly after their son was admitted to Children's Hospital. Shortly after his parents were informed that Oliver had died, they remembered being asked by a young female doctor if they wished to sign an organ donor permission. However, they were certain she had told them that only eyes and skin could be donated. NICU staff confirmed that this standard organ donor consent form was routinely provided to the parents and guardians of all admissions to the Children's NICU who died. It was not consent for surgery and was restricted to research using cells from the eyes and skin.

None of the members of the cleaning staff caught in the raid spoke English. Through an interpreter, they explained in Arabic that they were dropped off outside the loading dock every evening at nine p.m., entering the transplant unit through the front entrance of the research building and subsequently, according to gender, accessing the transplant unit by way of the male or female restrooms. The process was reversed in the morning at four a.m.

Drs. Daher and Sula, who were not arrested at the scene but reportedly visited the transplant unit regularly to see patients, both separately asserted that they are Saudi Arabian citizens and Dr. Paul Kader has threatened them and their families. Kader has disappeared, along with his wife, her mother, and their five children. None of his household staff has seen any of them since the evening prior to the police raid. There is preliminary evidence that the family has left the country and are now in Pakistan. Dr. Daher and the Nurse Director of the South Baltimore NICU have both been interrogated and released under surveillance, having surrendered their passports.

Of the other suspects, Don Evans strikes me as a weak link and a transparent liar. However, he has stuck to his claim that he had no knowledge of the existence of the transplant unit.

Any heartening aspects of the case relate to the rescued infants. Both Oliver Turner and the other infant who was presumably destined to be a heart donor are doing well and, according to Dr. Sim, neither show evidence of residual damage from their experiences to date. Oliver Turner is at home; the other infant has been placed in foster care until his parents can be traced.

The post-transplant infant is apparently doing well, but his heart donor – that poor baby – we've found no trace of his identity, let alone his parents. And I can't charge Christian Carter with murder without an identified victim.

The infant who was to have received Oliver Turner's heart on the day of the raid remains in critical condition. Transplant unit staff have informed us that the parents of this infant are not in the United States. They think that his parents are Saudi Arabian but claim to have been provided with no identifying information other than initials. The Saudi Embassy has been asked to assist in the search for the parents of this critically ill infant whose clinical management has become a crisis for the Medical Ethics Committee at Children's Hospital. In the absence of his parents, a lay Guardian ad Litem has been court appointed to make surrogate decisions regarding his care. Placed in an unenviable position, the Guardian will need a great deal of support.

Dr. Sim explained to me that the Ethics Committee members had first to reach a consensus regarding whether to proceed with the standard palliative shunt surgery for his heart defect, the only choice in the absence of a donor's heart, or to place him on end-of-life care on the basis that he has already suffered irreversible organ damage. I haven't heard anything from the Saudi Embassy, and it remains unclear whether there are unknown conspirators among the employees at Children's Hospital. If I can't persuade Christian Carter to provide the names and contact information for the missing parents, I'll ask Dr. Sim for advice on this issue.

Sylvia stood up, carried her mug out of her office to the sink in the staff lounge, smoothed her skirt, and made her way to Interrogation Room Five.

Awaiting her in the small, windowless room were Dr. Christian Carter, his lawyer, and Lieutenant Strand.

Carter had paid the sizeable bail set by the judge and was impeccably dressed in a dark blue suit that matched his eyes. He was sitting rigidly upright with an expressionless face. Sylvia was aware that there were four observers on the other side of the one-way mirror.

"Good afternoon, Dr. Carter."

As she took a seat at the table, opposite Carter, and reached over to turn on the recording machine, Sylvia nodded to his well-preserved, blond, middle-aged female lawyer. "It is three minutes past fifteen hundred hours, on Tuesday, March third, nineteen eighty-seven. This is the second interrogation of Dr. Christian Lee Carter. In the room are Colonel Sylvia Parker and Lieutenant Strand, Baltimore City Police, and Ms. Rebecca Cohen, representing Dr. Carter."

Sylvia leaned across the table toward Christian Carter and looked him in the eyes. "Dr. Carter, when you completed medical school did you take the Hippocratic Oath or something equivalent?"

"Yes. It wasn't required but I did take it."

"Would you agree that the Hippocratic Oath emphasizes the sanctity of the doctor-patient relationship and requires that the doctor not inflict unavoidable injury on their patient?"

"Yes. That's a reasonable synopsis."

"Then, doctor, I'm going to ask you to help us to trace the parents of the infants who were admitted to the heart transplant unit at South Baltimore Community Hospital from the date that it opened. You will surely agree that this is the least you can do to address the harm you have done to these infants and their families?"

Carter responded without any sign of emotion. "I certainly do not agree. I have spent my career attempting to cure babies with deadly heart conditions. I hear that the infant I transplanted recently is doing well and has a good prognosis. In my opinion, it is you and your colleagues who should search their conscience. You have prevented a critically ill infant from having his faulty heart replaced. He should also be doing well, but instead, he will probably die."

Despite herself, Sylvia Parker suffered a pang of guilt; she quickly recovered. "Do you agree that the murder of a human being to save the life of another human being is never ethically justified?"

"I strongly object to your use of the word 'murder'. Parental consent was obtained for the donor infants, all of whom had been diagnosed as having severe brain damage that would not permit them to lead a normal life."

"How do you explain the fact that no signed surgical consent forms for either the heart donors or recipients have been located to date?"

"I cannot be held responsible for ensuring that documents are filed correctly. I'm head of a large team and a busy surgeon."

Sylvia attempted to regain eye contact with Carter, but he avoided her gaze. "Would you list for us before you leave today, Dr. Carter, the members of your *large* team who are responsible for filing important documents like consent forms? And, in the meantime, in lieu of the consent forms, we ask that you provide us, through your legal representative Ms. Cohen, with parental contact information for all infants admitted to the transplant unit apart from Oliver Turner."

For the first time since the interrogation began, Christian Carter's face lost its disdainful expression. Beads of sweat were forming on his upper lip and forehead. He leaned close to Ms. Cohen and whispered behind his hand.

"I'd like to confer with my client alone, Colonel." Said, Ms. Cohen.

Ten minutes later they were all back in the interrogation room. As soon as the recorder was turned on and the recommencement data recorded, Ms. Cohen stated for the record. "My client invokes the Fifth Amendment, specifically as it applies to the right of an individual not to serve as a witness in a criminal case in which they are the defendant."

Chapter 19

Saturday, March 14th, 1987, 4:30 p.m.

DRESSED IN STREET CLOTHES, COLONEL PARKER WAS deep in conversation with Lussi, seated on a bench in a small, enclosed grassy area behind the Central Baltimore Police Headquarters. A light rain was falling.

The Colonel, although speaking softly, was gesticulating with uncharacteristic intensity. "…it's frustrating that this children's toy, which probably has nothing to do with the case, is the only thing found at the site that our forensics team is certain is the one from which both shots were fired at Bill Shultz. Everything else found there clearly predated the shooting.

"More aggravating is the claim of jurisdiction that the CIA has just placed on the case after we've done most of the heavy lifting. Our hands are tied because the international aspects of the matter legitimize their involvement."

"What does this mean for the people who have already given statements? Will the CIA interview everyone again? That seems a colossal waste of time."

"No, Doctor, I'm sure that they will re-interrogate only selected suspects, as we're now doing, but they won't bother with others unless they are perceived as a weak link whom they can coerce into 'ratting' on someone else. However, the fact that the CIA is so emphatic about being in charge, rather than simply cooperating, does arouse a concern for me that some of their own agents may be involved in *Broken Hearts*, and they don't want them exposed. After all, we now know that Bill Schultz was working for them."

"How do you know this about Bill Schultz? Do you mean the CIA has been aware that he was involved in this conspiracy for some time?"

"Yes, I'm afraid so and this isn't unprecedented. If there's an international 'situation' that the CIA perceive can be manipulated to serve the 'best interests of the United States,' they will place their agents on one or multiple sides of the operation. We know about Schultz because Don Evans finally broke under interrogation today. He was offered a plea deal by the federal prosecutor and took it without hesitation. He has confirmed that Bill informed him that he worked for the CIA, and that Bill was the key liaison with the Saudis, responsible for the American end of all funding arrangements for South Baltimore Community Hospital. Don also revealed that the Saudi family who donated the funds for a cardiac research unit are members of the Saudi royal family, as is Dr. Paul Kader."

"Whoa – how long has the CIA been watching this case evolve, Colonel? Are you saying that they have known that the *situation*, as you call it, involved infanticide, and yet decided not to intervene?"

"No, frankly I don't think they knew about the heart transplant unit. I gather they are following an international financial trail, involving some of their '*usual suspects*,' and have assumed, up to now, that all the money involved is used to purchase weapons.

"However, speaking of those infants, I'm hoping that you might provide me with substantial assistance. I'll be completely candid with you, the request I'm going to make is far from standard police procedure, but *Broken Hearts* is far from a standard case. This murderous bunch must be rapidly brought to justice and, to achieve this end, I am more than willing to put my job on the line. I ask that you listen to all I am about to say before responding. Is that OK with you?"

"Yes – I guess so."

"Doctor, I perceive that you are a person of genuine integrity, dedicated to providing the best possible care to your patients. You have certainly demonstrated that you are both courageous and resourceful. Knowing this about you, I don't want to put you in a situation that you cannot refuse and, thus, place you in additional danger.

"Having said this, the murder of Bill Schultz has made it likely that, in addition to Schultz and Carter, there are personnel at Children's Hospital who are involved in the *Broken Hearts* conspiracy but remain under our radar. I have reached the point when my gut tells me you are the only person that I can rely on for valid inside information regarding possible suspects.

"We agreed last weekend that the press would be notified that you are no longer a missing person, and that seems to have gone smoothly. You have told me you plan to return to work on the twenty-third. I predict you will be greeted as a celebrity and, having got to know you a little, I think your inclination will be to hide in the NICU. I am asking you to do the opposite – without displaying behavior that is out of character, but being on the alert for anything that seems out-of-line. Most urgently, I need to discover the identities of conspirators at Children's and figure out how Oliver Turner became a victim. I had hoped that Christian Carter might have retained some remnants of conscience and would provide me with information on the identities and origins of the other two donor infants, but instead, he immediately took the 'fifth'. I have asked the CIA to help, but I don't get the feeling it is a priority for them. Do you know of any international children's agencies who might help us out, doctor?"

"I wish I did, colonel. Fortunately, I have never encountered a situation like this before. Let me think about it and do some research."

"Remember doctor, the number one mandate for this undertaking is that you *do not* take any risks or confront anyone. You have access to patient data at Children's, and I will provide you with patient files and other pertinent data confiscated from South Baltimore Hospital. What are your thoughts?"

"Well, I'm not looking forward to fielding all the likely questions when I return to work, but I do want to help you, and am confident that I can do so without drawing attention to myself."

"Doctor, my concern is not that you will fail to achieve what you set out to do, but that you will allow your passion to overtake your caution. You are a known adversary to these people, so they will be on the alert, and you will have to be exquisitely careful not to arouse suspicion that you are doing anything other than your job.

"Your home may still be bugged. It is unlikely because we've searched, found, and removed several bugs, but not impossible – so please don't discuss *Broken Hearts* at home. I think the safest way for us to communicate is for me to lend you a mobile police phone. They are quite bulky but would fit in your briefcase. Also, I think it is time we were on first-name terms, so how about you adopt a new one for the purposes of communication? How about your name becoming 'Carole'? If you call me, suggest a friendly get-together. If you leave a message, leave it for 'Sara' – you can assume I will respond appropriately. In the reverse, I'll call you daily to check in at a prearranged time when you are out of earshot – perhaps in your car?"

"I could best answer your calls during my drive to work in the morning because I leave home at pretty much the same time every day. When I'm on call overnight it could screw us up a little, but I will get a copy of my on-call schedule to you."

"That sounds fine, 'Carole' – we have time to refine the plan before your return to work, and I suggest we decide on an initial emergency meeting place in advance so that there is no risk of revealing it during a call."

"Thumbs up to that Colonel."

"Hold on 'Carole' – from now on you will address me only as 'Sara'. This way, if you call me in a difficult place to talk, I'll inform you that you have the wrong number and call you back.

"Also, there's something else you need to know. Suzanne Sinclair has disappeared. We have no evidence that she's left Baltimore, but no one in the Sinclair household, including her husband, the housekeeper, and the stable hands admit to having any idea where she might be. The odd thing is, when I talked to her on the night Bill Schultz was shot, she struck me as honest, smart, and attempting to be helpful. We have, to date, found no evidence that she was involved in *Broken Hearts*."

"Her poor husband must be distraught. George adores Suzanne."

"Donna Schultz said much the same thing. Although clearly ignorant of her husband's clandestine activities, she revealed that she was fully aware that Bill and Suzanne Sinclair had been having an affair since before Bill and she moved from Houston to Baltimore. She regretted not informing George about the affair, but she said he was so obviously blinded by love for his wife, she hadn't the heart to shatter his illusions. Donna admitted that she had long accepted her husband for what he was, and simply wanted a peaceful life."

"It is a relief to me to hear that Donna knew about the affair. I've felt guilty knowing about it but saying nothing."

"Well, to get back to our plan. I will, of course, continue the police presence outside your home, and protection will be extended to cover your drive to and from the hospital. But I can't protect you inside the hospital, so you *must* be extremely careful. Tomorrow, I will meet you at the place and time previously discussed."

"Heard and understood, Sara. I am grateful for the opportunity to help."

Chapter 20

Monday, March 23rd, 1987, 8:00 a.m.

Lussi dreaded returning to work, but it proved anticlimactic. Barbara and the other office staff welcomed her warmly and didn't ask questions. Her medical colleagues, with the notable exception of Azad Sula, who had been suspended from work pending the conclusion of the investigation into his role in *Broken Hearts*, showed her the same consideration.

After NICU rounds, on the way to radiology to review X-rays with the team, Lussi encountered Joe Meridian as he was about to enter the cardiac catheterization laboratory.

Joe did a doubletake, stopped in his tracks, strode over to Lussi, and enveloped her in his arms. "Lussi, welcome back! I've really missed you. Are you OK?" Taking Lussi by the shoulders, he pushed her away from him a little and scrutinized her face. "You look tired."

Lussi smiled, catching her breath from the hug. "Hi Joe, I'm fine. Happy to be back. I'm due in imaging rounds now but do want to thank you for all the support you've given Ann Castle and the others while I've been away. Your ears should have been burning with all the compliments they've given you."

"I was happy to do it. What would we do without the NICU staff?" Joe reached out and gently patted the back of Lussi's head. "How are you doing? Any residual effects?"

"No, I'm perfectly fine I'm happy to say."

"Well, that's great Lussi. They're waiting for me to do a catheterization, so I must get going, but let's catch up later over a cup of coffee."

Lussi smiled and gave Joe a thumbs-up as she turned to follow her team to the Imaging Suite.

Keeping Colonel Parker's request in mind, Lussi forced herself to go to the cafeteria for lunch. It had become her habit over recent years to eat in her office. She valued the time to herself, no matter how brief, but had to acknowledge that she'd missed out on a lot of hospital gossip this way, some of which might, in retrospect, have been valuable. As she left the food line with her tray, she saw her colleague Mary Morrison sitting at a table with Sarah Gold, the Medical Director of the Blood Bank, and Alka Subramanian, the Director of Pathology. They waved her over to join them.

Lussi was greeted enthusiastically as she took her seat at the table. As expected, there were questions about her well-being, and it seemed general knowledge that she'd been kidnapped at South Baltimore Community Hospital and had played a key role in breaking up a corrupt enterprise there. Lussi managed to field these questions without providing additional information.

During lunch, Lussi learned that with no charges having been filed against her, the hospital Board had appointed Sherry Dunstan as acting Chief Operating Officer. This appointment was not popular with Children's Hospital employees. The NICU at South Baltimore had been closed by the Maryland State Health authorities. No obstetric services would be provided there until further notice.

Mary Morrison listed five or six people who stood out for their support and assistance while Lussi was away. The list was headed by Ann Castle and Joe Meridian.

"Joe's willingness to pitch in and help is impressive," Mary told her. "He even volunteered to take on the massive job of digging through all research protocols approved by the Institutional Research Committee over the past two years, on top of all his other responsibilities. Joe's wife must be unselfish – he always seems to be at work."

Lussi didn't share with Mary her own impression of Joe's wife. Unselfish wasn't the description that came to mind. "Imperious" was closer to the mark.

As Lussi stood up to leave, Alka grasped her hand. "It's so great to have you back, Lussi, and I'm sorry to bring this up so soon after your return, but when would it be convenient for us to discuss a couple of concerns relating to the attendance of your fellows at autopsies?"

"Darn it, that doesn't sound good, Alka. I have emphasized to them that attending autopsies on their patients is an invaluable learning experience that they cannot afford to miss. How about two p.m. tomorrow in your office?"

"That will be fine and don't worry Lucy, these issues will be easily resolved."

Lussi blessed her good luck. She had intended to call Alka this afternoon to request a meeting, so their lunchtime encounter was fortuitous. She was, of course, concerned that her fellows might not be attending autopsies as they should be, but the meeting with Alka also offered Lussi the opportunity to ask her for her help with the question of how it had been possible to declare Oliver Turner dead, deposit his body in the pathology department, then remove him alive from the hospital?

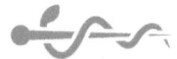

5:35 p.m.

THERE WERE FEW PEOPLE IN THE HOSPITAL CAFETERIA at this time of day; too late for those going home and too early for those remaining in the hospital overnight. Joe was sitting alone at a relatively secluded table in a corner of the dining room. Only one cash register was open, and from the kitchen issued sounds indicative of large-scale dishwashing.

As she approached Joe's table, Lussi saw two cups of untouched coffee on the table in front of Joe and, when he looked up to greet her, she was struck by the shadows under his eyes. In place of his usual exemplary posture, his body was slumped in the seat. His coat and briefcase were on the seat opposite him.

Joe smiled, patting the chair beside him, and pushing a cup of coffee in Lussi's direction. "I know that I've already said this, probably several times, but it's so great to have you back, Lussi. I really have missed you, and not only because you're the only one who appreciates my jokes. But seriously, I can't imagine what you have been through."

"One of these days I'll feel I can talk about it, Joe, but right now I don't want to relive any of it. I hope you understand."

"I absolutely appreciate how you feel, Lussi. As you can imagine, things have been chaotic since the discovery at South Baltimore. I am embarrassed that I had no idea what was going on there, even though I've worked closely with Christian Carter for several years. I mean, I always knew he had a sizeable ego, and it was obvious he was really pissed-off when the transplant program here was terminated, but he is a bright guy and a good surgeon. What on earth was he thinking?"

"Well, you sat next to me at Christian's last presentation at Grand Rounds, Joe. Remember – when he was pushing the idea of improving the prognosis for babies with hypoplastic left heart syndrome by skipping the shunt procedure and performing heart transplantation soon after birth? I must admit that I was caught up in his enthusiasm because you know how I feel about the long wait for a compatible heart, while the infant develops a damaging infection or irreversible side effects from supportive treatment. You and I discussed his hypothesis at the time, and we agreed that an earlier transplant might be the right way to go, were we living in a parallel universe where there was a ready supply of transplantable infant hearts. I guess the opportunity to test his hypothesis totally unfettered by ethical restrictions overcame any reservations Christian might have."

"Relative to ethical considerations, Lussi, I discovered that Christian did in fact submit a research proposal to the research committee. He proposed performing fetal surgery on in-utero piglets so that they were born with a heart defect comparable to a hypoplastic left heart in humans. Then, within the first two weeks of life, he was going to transplant normal piglet donor hearts into a randomly selected fifty percent of the piglets born with the heart defect. He intended to perform standard palliative shunt surgery on the other fifty percent and provide them with long-term intensive care support, prior to transplanting a normal piglet heart at age six to eight months, depending on their weight. It was a well-designed research project, and it was approved by the Institutional Research Committee, but it would have taken several years to complete, and even then, as you know so well, two major problems remain. Findings in an animal model can't be directly applied to humans and, even if he clearly showed improved outcome in the cohort of piglets undergoing early heart transplant, where would he get the infant donor hearts to test this result in human infants?"

Lussi was puzzled. *I've been a member of the research committee for the past three years and I rarely miss a meeting, but I'm certain I've never reviewed this protocol, let alone voted for approval.*

"Yes, Joe. I heard that you've volunteered to review all IRC protocols submitted in the past two years. That's a mammoth undertaking. Can you remember when Christian's protocol was reviewed?"

"Yes actually, I can. It struck me as strange that you would not have mentioned it to me, but then I double-checked and confirmed that it was reviewed at the January meeting this year, while you were away in Norway. As for extra work Lussi, the job isn't nearly as onerous as it sounds. I've only been asked to review protocols that are in any way related to cardiac surgery and, I must admit, from the aspect of research productivity, in the past twenty-four months there hasn't been a huge number of research protocols presented to the IRC by a principal investigator in the cardiac surgery division. In comparison to them, our division is productive, and your division excels."

"That's nice of you to say, Joe."

"Well, I've always believed in interdisciplinary cooperation rather than competition. I wish all our colleagues felt the same."

Interdisciplinary cooperation, that's what I need to fulfill the responsibility the Colonel has given me – I need Joe's expertise to help me answer this question. If I can't trust him, who can I trust?

Moral Injury

"Joe, have you figured out how Oliver Turner was declared dead and processed through pathology when he was actually still alive?"

Joe stopped smiling. "No, sadly I haven't Lussi. It was made *very* clear to all of us when we were questioned by the police that they would do the investigating and we were to stay out of it. I was asked if I'd any idea how it could have been done, and I told them I didn't have the faintest idea because Alka maintains an admirably tight ship in Pathology."

"Yes, that is the factor that makes this so impossible to figure out Joe. I'm going to meet with Alka and see if we can come up with any answers."

Joe's eyebrows rose. "Lussi, please let the police do their work. You've done enough and got yourself kidnapped in the process. Besides, Azad Sula was responsible for Oliver Turner's care the day he died, and the police have him in custody. Surely, he must know how it happened."

Oh God, I'm doing exactly what the Colonel warned me against.

"You are quite right, Joe." Lussi hoped her sigh of capitulation was not overdone. "I understand where you're coming from, and I appreciate your concern. Best to allow the police to do their job." She smiled at Joe and drained her coffee cup. "Thanks for the coffee, Joe. You look exhausted and I have quite a bit of work to finish before I go home, so I had better get going."

As she stood, reaching for her empty coffee cup, Joe caught Lussi's arm, guiding her back onto her seat.

Sotto voce, Joe said, "Lussi, forgive me for coming over a bit strong but I care about your safety. The police have emphatically warned us not to investigate on our own. You, of all people, should be aware of the dangers of snooping, quite apart from the possibility that you may impede police efforts to solve the case and get Alka in trouble to boot.

"Jesus, here I go again bullying you. Please do forgive me. Like just about everyone else on staff here, I feel quite stressed by this shocking mess at South Baltimore."

Lussi was touched by Joe's investment in the role of her protector; her instincts told her not to argue. She stood and put a hand on his.

"There is nothing to forgive, Joe. I'm grateful that you are concerned about my safety, and you are right; I should know better."

"Thank you, Lussi; gracious as always."

Lussi smiled. "I'll talk to you tomorrow."

Joe followed Lussi out of the cafeteria and turned in the direction of the main lobby. Lussi headed to her office to collect her coat and briefcase.

Chapter 21

Tuesday, March 24th, 1987, 1:55 p.m.

For her meeting with Alka Subramanian, Lussi took a circuitous route to Pathology. This entailed leaving the hospital and reentering through a door near the hospital incinerator. She checked repeatedly to make sure she was not being followed.

As soon as Lussi entered her office, Alka handed her a mug of coffee. They sat down at a circular table that held three double-headed microscopes and several boxes of glass slides.

"Before we get started," said Alka, "I want to tell you that the reason I asked you to meet with me has nothing to do with the attendance record of your fellows at autopsies. In fact, your fellows are role models for the trainees on other services. I just wanted that out of the way in case I'd caused you any anxiety. I need to talk to you about a problem I'm not sure how to deal with. I would value your help greatly, but please keep what I'm about to say strictly between us."

Lussi breathed a sigh of relief. "I have a feeling we both want to talk about the same thing, Alka. Does this have anything to do with the investigation at South Baltimore Hospital?"

"Absolutely. I've been questioned twice by the police. It was all very friendly but centered around the procedure involved in signing a dead patient into and out of our department. Obviously, I don't know the details of what went on at South Baltimore, but I gather that the police believe that at least one infant died, and they are trying to trace his origin. The police informed me that it is possible that the baby was stolen from a family, rather than a hospital, but no missing baby has been reported in the past six months within a hundred-mile radius of the Baltimore beltway.

"Then there is the question of the Turner baby. All the standard morgue paperwork is in place for him. How was a live infant admitted to and then discharged from my department? This should not be possible and is the reason why the police suspect that at least one of my staff must have been involved. I have worked for years with the staff members who signed baby Turner in and out of the morgue and, personally, have no doubts about their integrity. But they are both being treated as suspects by the police."

"These questions are exactly what I need to discuss with you, Alka. Before we start, how much did the police tell you about what was going on at South Baltimore or what happened to me?"

"Well, just the bare bones – that there was an illegal heart transplant unit over there and there was evidence that a baby had died. They didn't mention you at all and they did not encourage me to ask questions. They did make it clear that I must not discuss the case with anyone."

"Thanks, Alka."

Lussi stood, walked over to a whiteboard, and picked up a marker. "Alka, I'm a visual thinker, so I'm going to diagram an average timeline for dealing with Oliver Turner's 'remains' in the NICU, and then would you do the same thing for the standard procedure in Pathology?"

Lussi drew and talked, indicating that, since Oliver's parents didn't want an autopsy, the airway tube and all lines could be removed by the nurses. However, because Oliver's "death" had occurred within seventy-two hours of his admission to the NICU, Dr. Sula or the neonatology fellow should have called the Medical Examiner's Office to determine whether an autopsy was mandatory. The ME's decision should then have been recorded in the patient chart and, if an autopsy was deemed mandatory, the ME's decision would override parental wishes and all tubes and lines would remain in place in the body.

"I called the ME's office and confirmed that Dr. Sula did call them about the autopsy, Alka. It was not deemed a case for their office, on the grounds that Oliver was so critically ill when he was admitted to the NICU that there was nothing unexpected about his death."

Alka nodded. "That sounds like a reasonable response from them in the circumstances."

Lussi put down the marker and spoke her thoughts out loud. "Now – *there is* a way that a full pathology admission-discharge process might have been bypassed. By falsely claiming that Oliver was an ME's case?"

"Well, no Lussi, the body would still have to be processed through our department. Besides, as I said, all the correct paperwork is in place. Shall I take over now and map out a timeline for processing bodies into and out of our morgue?"

Alka continued Lussi's diagram, indicating the role and average time taken by clerical and other staff to record the arrival time of the body, ensure that all required paperwork and the hospital records were complete, and prepare for and place Oliver's body into the freezer. These procedures added approximately thirty minutes to Lussi's timeline.

"Do you keep a record of any of the key points in your timeline for each case, Alka?"

"We record the time of arrival in pathology, but not the time that the body is placed in the freezer, although I'm thinking of making the latter a requirement in the future. But, to tell you the truth, in all the years I've practiced pathology in the States, I've not encountered a case like this. It was very different in Pakistan, where I went to medical school; there, bodies got lost all the time."

"Alka, once a body is in the freezer, and I'm assuming that Oliver Turner's body was put there, how long do they usually remain if there is not going to be an autopsy?"

"That's very variable, Lussi, especially for a morgue in a hospital serving an inner-city population as we do. Sadly, we not infrequently have cases where the body is never picked up and, after a certain period, we incinerate them."

"So how long, approximately, do you think Oliver's body was in the freezer? The kidnappers surely could not risk leaving a live baby in there for long."

"Lussi, that is a problematic aspect of our handling of Oliver's body. The record indicates that Oliver was to be placed in freezer two, slot twenty-one, but there is no evidence that this happened. When I spoke to the staff that were on duty that day, they told me that the hearse from the funeral home arrived while they were still completing the paperwork on Oliver, so that he was discharged prior to placement in the freezer. One of my staff said that the man from the funeral home told him that one of the doctors at Children's was paying for the funeral and requested that they pick up Oliver's body as soon as possible."

"He didn't give the name of the doctor?"

"Unfortunately, no. Our guy had the impression that the man from the funeral home didn't know."

Lussi took a sip of coffee. "What if we hypothesize that the body taken to pathology was not Oliver's? I can't believe that the kidnappers would want to risk damaging their heart donor by placing him in a freezer for even a short time, and I'm certain your staff would immediately recognize that an infant was sedated rather than deceased. The NICU identification bracelets stay on the dead infants – they must have put Oliver's bracelets on a dead baby and somehow snuck Oliver out of the NICU."

"Well Lussi, I've checked and double-checked all the bodies in the morgue, and none are missing or unidentified. In addition, no other infant died in the hospital on the day that Oliver was removed from ECMO."

"I'm very grateful to you for all this helpful information, Alka. Sadly, I think that the police are correct – there are likely to have been more infants murdered than just the one donor infant that we know about. I'll think over what we've discussed and let you know if I come up with any additional thoughts."

"I should be thanking you, Lussi. There is just one more thing. Regarding the possible source of the unidentified heart donor, the police let it drop, either intentionally or by accident, that there were a significant number of Saudi Arabians working at South Baltimore Hospital. I was born in Pakistan. The Muslims in Pakistan and in Saudi Arabia are under Sharia Law. Sharia Law in the strictest interpretation, which I know is the case in Saudi Arabia, does not allow adoption. I've a feeling that abandoned babies might not be too difficult to procure from orphanages in Saudi Arabia without questions being asked."

Lussi retraced her steps to her office, shocked by the implications of Alka's parting words.

7:30 p.m.

As it turned out, Colonel Parker and Lussi had to use their communication plan faster than either of them anticipated.

Arriving almost simultaneously in separate taxis, they were shown to a table at a restaurant in Little Italy.

A Puccini opera was playing from speakers above their dimly lit alcove.

"Are you certain that no one followed you here?" asked the Colonel.

She had kept her eyes trained on the restaurant entrance since they sat down.

"Yes, I followed your instructions precisely, Sara. I first drove back to Children's from home, with your guys following. I left my car in the garage and used a phone in the hospital atrium to call a cab. I did not see anyone I knew. The cab picked me up at an entrance at the rear of the hospital. I shall reverse the route on the way back."

There was a pause while a waiter took their drink order.

"Where does your husband believe you are?"

"I told him the truth. I was more than halfway home when you called me on the police mobile, and Howard arrived home shortly after I did. I handed him a note telling him I was meeting you but did not give him the location. He assumed that the meeting was to be at your office. I'm sorry, but I just couldn't bring myself to lie to Howard. He was concerned about me driving alone, but I explained that you had assigned police officers to follow me."

At that moment, a waiter brought their drinks. Lussi took a sip of her wine and there was another pause while they ordered their food.

Lussi expected to be admonished for failure to follow instructions. Instead, the Colonel said quietly, "Carole, I contacted you because, since we last spoke, I have received information from my liaison in the CIA that has caused me to rethink my approach to certain aspects of *Broken Hearts*. We must discuss and resolve some urgent issues."

Lussi put down her wine glass and stared at the Colonel with raised eyebrows. "Has there been another murder?"

"Not that we know about. However, as you are aware, it is general knowledge among the executives and a significant number of the hospital staff at Children's Hospital that Suzanne Sinclair and Bill Schultz were having an affair. I bring this up again now because Suzanne remains a missing person of interest, we have no solid leads to her possible whereabouts, and her husband George now appears to be one of the few people I've interviewed in this case who was not aware of the affair. This makes me question his candor and wonder if I should look at him more closely for the murder of Bill Shultz. Could anyone really be as blind to what was going on around them as he claims he was?"

"Yes, emphatically, Sara There is no question in my mind that George had no idea what was going on between Suzanne and Bill Schultz. The rumor mill at Children's is vigorous and far-reaching. Bill and Suzanne made no attempt to be discreet – openly arriving together in the morning and leaving together at the end of the day. Since Bill brought Suzanne with him from Texas as his COO, and they had worked at the same hospital there, putting two and two together was easy for staff on the fifth floor. Rumors involving senior management tend to spread rapidly in a hospital.

"George is a relatively rare visitor to the hospital. When he does visit, he prefers to spend his time in the wards with the children. At Christmas time he does Santa Clause duties, and he is a substantial donor. I find him a wise, kind, and empathic man who, I am certain, would be a real asset to the hospital Board of Trustees if it weren't for the potential conflict-of-interest that he is married to the CFO. I just can't imagine George Sinclair hurting anyone. I thought you were about to charge Tony Blake with Bill's murder."

"Well Carole, I hope, if I'm ever in serious trouble, someone will give me a heartfelt testimonial like the one you just gave George Sinclair. Yes, Tony Blake has all the qualifications to be the chief suspect for Bill's murder, but alas, we can't disprove his alibi. He says he met his wife for dinner that evening at around seven p.m. and his wife, the two friends who joined them, and the waiter who served them have all backed him up. Of course, in view of his unprepossessing personality, I haven't ruled out the possibility that he hired a hitman.

"To get back on track, since I spoke to you last, I've received more information from the CIA on Bill Schultz. Apparently, Bill spent part of his youth in Saudi Arabia and Tunisia while his father was *chargé d' affairs* for the United States Embassy in Saudi Arabia. He went to school with Saudi princes, making close friendships with many of them. Bill's wife says that he loved the affluent lifestyle, became an excellent polo player, and studied Arabic in Tunisia, before returning to the United States to earn his MBA."

"Saudi Arabia, where the donation for the cardiac surgery research unit came from."

And it fits with the horrifying suggestion that Alka made this afternoon.

"Yes, both South Baltimore Hospital and the heart transplant unit appear to have been developed using money that originated there." The Colonel paused while the waiter served their entrees.

The restaurant was filling up and the noise level was almost drowning the Italian opera. Lussi stared at her food – she had no appetite.

"Can you at least pretend that you are enjoying your meal, Carole? No one should overhear us here, but I wouldn't want to encourage anyone to try." The Colonel handed Lussi a fork. "It is a long story, so please plan to order dessert and coffee."

Lussi managed to smile and began to pick at her food.

"At some point before he and Donna were married, Bill was recruited by the CIA. I'm informed by my resource that, at the time of Bill's recruitment, CIA finances were strained, and the Saudi royal family's petrochemical dollars were a very attractive financial source for CIA-backed covert interventions in the Middle East. Bill's access to high-ranking members of the royal family played a key role in setting up a money laundering program for the CIA. The Saudis sent the money to their embassy in Washington. The Saudi ambassador in Washington then transferred the money to a Swiss bank account controlled by the CIA. The CIA used that account to make covert purchases on the international arms market."

Lussi interrupted, "So how did Bill end up as a hospital CEO?"

"Well, over time, the United States' alliance with Saudi Arabia has become all about fighting communism. The Russians support Marxists and nationalist movements in the Middle East. The Saudis saw the Russian ingress into Afghanistan as the first step in a broader Soviet plan. The United States and the Saudis agreed to covertly ship weapons to the Afghan Mujahideen, who are fighting the government of Afghanistan and the Russians. Bill, with his MBA and high-ranking Saudi friends, was perfect for the role of CIA facilitator.

"The Saudis had already provided over two billion dollars to the Mujahideen war effort when uncomfortable questions started to be asked in Congress, and President Reagan needed to hide the role of the United States in the Afghanistan war. So, while Congress was steadfastly refusing to permit large-scale weapons sales to the Arab world, coincidentally Saudi annual oil income decreased from around one hundred billion dollars to about twenty billion dollars. In response to the resulting decrease in Saudi funding, Bill and others were instructed by the CIA to devise new laundering schemes that involved investment in commercial enterprises that promised to generate profit on the money. By this juncture, Bill knows his way around the for-profit healthcare industry, hence the decision to build South Baltimore Hospital. However, my CIA contact is adamant that the transplant unit was not part of Bill's assigned mission.

Lussi put down her fork and leaned back in her seat with a sigh. "It sounds like a movie script; I can't make it seem real."

"You haven't heard all of it, Carole – as the amount they are paid for oil decreases, the Saudi royal family's size and lifestyle continue to cost so much that their bank accounts are shrinking. They also have lots of children; some Princes have as many as seventy. As a result, there are more than twenty-thousand members of the Saudi royal family, and they are all living in luxury."

"So, just to be clear, Sara, financial circumstances for the Saudi royal family are deteriorating and, coincidentally, Congress puts the brakes on the sale of weapons to Arab countries. Now, I guess Bill's underhand expertise is in even greater demand?" Lussi observed.

"Absolutely, Carole. From the start, the Saudis have categorized as 'off budget spending' the funds that they assign to purchase weapons for the Mujahideen. The money goes directly into special accounts, bypassing the Saudi Treasury, and is used to pay for 'special projects' with no government audits or accountability. Enormous commissions and bribes are required to complete these projects. Desperate to maintain their indulgent lifestyle, some members of the royal family have developed shady business practices both in Saudi Arabia and the United States, and Bill, it seems, was ready and willing to assist them.

"By the time he became CEO of Children's Hospital, Bill was retired from active fieldwork with the CIA. He was concentrating on maintaining and personally profiting from the flow of Saudi money, both through money laundering and through the United States stock market, where billions of dollars are deposited by members of the Saudi royal family. Bill also assisted the Saudis with collecting bribes from construction firms, seeking government contracts, setting up international arms deals, and even selling visas to guest workers. I am informed that he probably learned these 'off the books' techniques from Mob connections he developed during CIA undercover operations."

"The Mob? Maybe they put out a hit on him?"

"Believe me, we are including that possibility in our investigations and also the possibility that the Saudis had him killed to shut him up."

Lussi frowned. "I can't understand why Bill came to Children's rather than becoming CEO of South Baltimore Hospital?"

"We think that Bill took the precaution of having the Saudis hire Don Evans as 'puppet' CEO for South Baltimore Hospital so that he could physically distance himself from what was going on there and use the not-for-profit status of Children's Hospital to cloak illicit financial activities.

"This information I'm sharing with you opens new avenues for our murder investigation, which is positive for us but not the reason I am sharing it with you. I want you to understand the reasons behind the revised instructions I am about to give you.

"I was seriously remiss and went against acceptable police procedure when I asked you to collect information for me at your workplace. From the beginning, it has been clear that the perpetrators in this case are extremely dangerous, but I believed that the risks had significantly diminished after the raid. As we learn more about the major players in *Broken Hearts*, however, it has become quite clear that we are up against a highly sophisticated and depraved international network. I want you – no, I am ordering you to discontinue your investigatory activities immediately. Just keep a low profile at work from now on and let us do our job."

I am into this too far to quit. Sorry Colonel – I can't do what you ask.

As their waiter again approached the table, Lussi said quickly, "Thank you for your concern about my well-being, Sara. I quite understand." They both ordered dessert and coffee, then Lussi headed for the ladies' room.

I admire Sylvia Parker and don't like deceiving her, but there's no other way. I will have to put up some resistance when I get back to the table; she will be suspicious if I give in to her too easily. Thank goodness I haven't had the opportunity to tell her about the meeting with Alka. I must review Oliver Turner's medical records from the day that he died without further delay.

Chapter 22

Wednesday, March 25th, 1987, 2:15 a.m.

Lussi awoke abruptly from a nightmare. She lay shuddering in the dark beside Howard, who was deeply asleep.

The dream was so clear. I remember every detail. I'm standing in a muddy military trench dressed in surgical scrubs. The trench is strewn with the corpses of soldiers, each one lying beside a muck-spattered incubator. I am acutely aware that I am the last 'man' standing, thus, I have a duty to determine whether the incubators are occupied and, if so, attempt rescue. Yet, with each step, my feet are sucked deeper into the mud. Abruptly, like a gas flame igniting on a stove, the closest dead soldier gyrates to an upright position; a bloodstained crater is all that remains of the back of her skull.

"We trusted you." She shrieks – over, and over again. I know this soldier is someone I should recognize, but I don't. I make it to the incubator next to her – the mire now almost reaching my knees. Peering inside, I see a bundled infant – a halo of blood on the mattress beneath the head. I struggle to the next incubator, and the next, and the next. I find an identical corpse in each one.

As if from a distance, I hear myself scream, 'I swear I will not fail you again – I promise I will remember', as I fall backward into the mud. Then I'm awake, but the cries of the dead soldier echo in my head as I strive to recall a vital lost clue.

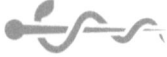

7 a.m.

Lussi paged Ann Castle, who responded immediately, reminding Lussi that she was staying overnight in a motel, close to the hospital in Southern Maryland where she was scheduled to lead an early morning workshop.

Lussi mentally chastised herself for not checking Ann's schedule. "Of course, now I remember, Ann. What time does the workshop begin? Do you have a couple of minutes?"

"Yes, I'm dressed and ready to go and we don't start until seven-thirty."

"I just need to check what time you are getting back to Children's. I'm going to look at Oliver Turner's patient chart to see if I can figure out how he was smuggled out of the hospital. Do you have time today to help me?"

"Sure do. I should be back around noon."

"Great – page me after you've had lunch."

On her way to morning rounds, Lussi stopped at Barbara's cubicle and asked her to call Medical Records to obtain the patient chart for Oliver Turner. Ten minutes into rounds, Barbara paged Lussi to tell her she would have to go down to Medical Records in person to review Oliver's chart. Because his patient file was part of a police investigation, it could not be removed from the records department.

As soon as rounds were over, Lussi went down to the medical records department in the hospital basement. Apart from the lady who delivered Oliver's file on a small cart, the place was empty. Lussi pushed the cart into one of the doorless cubicles provided for record review.

Despite the short duration of his hospitalization, Oliver's medical records were voluminous. Knowing that Ann would help her with the nursing records, Lussi extracted them from the file and put them aside. She began with the physicians' written notes. On the Friday prior to Oliver's "death", her last note in Oliver's chart was written at six twenty-five p.m. The note summarized Oliver's excellent progress and the content of her meeting with his parents. As was routine, a social worker had also attended this meeting. His note confirmed what Lussi had written.

The subsequent medical notes continued to document progressive improvement in Oliver's clinical status throughout Saturday. The last one for the day, written by a fellow, stated that the ECMO pump had been weaned to a low blood flow rate and a decision made, by Dr. Sula and the surgeon on call, that Oliver could be removed from ECMO the next day, following rounds. The fellow also noted that he'd called Oliver's parents to tell them the good news.

The earliest note for Sunday morning was written at six thirty by the senior surgical resident. He recorded plans to remove Oliver's ECMO cannulas at eleven a.m. At eight twenty there was a brief response to the surgical note, "Seen and appreciated." Signed by Dr. Sula. Subsequently, there were no other entries until two forty-eight p.m. when a final note was written and signed by Dr. Sula. In it, he stated that Oliver had been clinically stable when he rounded on him with the cardiology team at approximately eight-fifteen a.m., however, his condition had suddenly deteriorated while the cardiology team was in the ECMO room examining another patient. Oliver's blood pressure had fallen precipitously to dangerously low levels and the oxygen level in his blood also decreased, so that both his ventilator settings and the amount of oxygen provided required a significant increase.

When Dr. Sula arrived at Oliver's bedside for the second time that morning, he recorded that Dr. Meridian had his stethoscope on Oliver's chest and stated that Oliver had a heart murmur compatible with an open *ductus arteriosus*. Dr. Sula inserted a new IV needle and started an intravenous infusion of dopamine to treat Oliver's low blood pressure. Subsequently, a heart ultrasound and a chest X-ray confirmed that Oliver's *ductus arteriosus,* a blood vessel normally open only in the fetal state unless the newborn is premature or ill, had reopened and was causing right-sided heart failure. Oliver's parents were called and asked to come to the hospital as soon as possible. Resuscitation continued for a further thirty-five minutes before Oliver was pronounced dead. Oliver's parents arrived a few minutes later.

An addendum to this note, written half an hour later by Dr. Sula, was striking in its brevity. He didn't state who pronounced Oliver dead, the time of death, or detail his conversation with Oliver's parents, except to record that they did not wish an autopsy and had agreed to allow the hospital to cremate Oliver's body. He did record that the hospital chaplain was in the room and stayed to talk with Oliver's parents after he left.

I must talk to the chaplain.

Lussi thought a page must be missing from the record. She matched up the pages before and after Azad's note. The inadequate documentation appeared to be all there was. Azad had led her to believe that it was he who pronounced Oliver dead. This information should have been included in a detailed death note, with the time and date recorded.

Lussi now turned to the sheets recording Oliver's monitored physiologic data, including his ventilator settings, oxygen saturation of his blood, heart rate, blood pressure, urine output, and intravenous fluid intake. The forty-five minutes she spent scrutinizing these detailed notes produced no significant advance in her understanding of Oliver's clinical course, until she attempted to match the notes in the nursing and the medical records by the time of entry.

Working backward from Oliver's sudden decline, Lussi found information in the nursing record that either was missing from or differed significantly from the physician's notes. When the cardiology team had initially entered the ECMO room, they had rounded on Oliver first. Dr. Sula had not yet left for rounds in the NICU. Just before the cardiology team was recorded in the nursing notes as having moved on to examine the other ECMO patient, Oliver's nurse made a note that Dr. Sula was adjusting Oliver's ventilator settings.

This goes against NICU protocol. Physicians order ventilator changes but, unless it's an acute emergency, the changes are made and recorded by a respiratory therapist. At this point, Oliver's clinical status was described as "stable", so there was no indication to make changes to his ventilator settings.

A search of the respiratory therapy notes revealed no record of concurrent changes made by a respiratory therapist to Oliver's ventilator settings.

A wave of nausea hit Lussi.

Could Azad Sula have intentionally tampered with Oliver's ventilator to destabilize his clinical condition? But how could he then leave the ECMO room to do rounds in the NICU? Oliver was scheduled to be a live heart donor – why would Azad risk killing him or damaging his heart? The cardiologists were recorded in the nursing notes as arriving at the other ECMO patient's bedside only minutes before Azad left, so maybe he knew they would resuscitate Oliver.

No, this is crazy thinking – completely out of the realm of reality.

Her pager vibrated on the table. Using the phone on the cubical wall, Lussi told Ann she was in Medical Records.

Resuming her seat, her thoughts in turmoil, Lussi felt, rather than heard, a soft thud behind her. As she turned toward the cubical entrance, something sharp was pushed into the left side of her neck. She felt her upper body folding slowly toward the open file on the table but could do nothing to prevent it. From a far distance, she heard Barbara's voice. "I feel great sadness for this, Lussi. You were always good to me, but our *Cause* must come first. They tell me the dose of fentanyl is large; you will not feel any pain."

Then someone was shaking her, begging her to wake up.

Lussi struggled to speak. Using all the effort she could muster, she whispered, "Narcan."

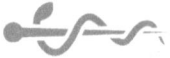

4.42 p.m.

"Well, hello, Dr. Lussi, I'm so happy to see your fingers moving."

Is someone inflating a tire? Who's up there?

"I'm Patty Weston, your primary nurse. You are in the Pediatric Intensive Care Unit at Children's Hospital. Don't try to talk – you are intubated and on a ventilator. Move your fingers again if you can hear me."

Fingers – yes.

"Mom, it's John, and Rachel's right beside me. Dad is talking to the police."

I can't breathe, I must breathe…. an alarm – someone's in trouble.

"Lussi dear, try to breathe with the ventilator; you are fighting it and setting off the alarm."

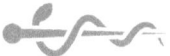

7.05 p.m.

Lussi took a sip of ice water to calm her burning throat and rasped a greeting to Sylvia Parker.

"Now I know how my patients feel."

Sylvia took a seat at the bedside and gazed at her. "I'm happy you are OK Lussi and grateful to you for agreeing to talk to me so soon after this dreadful assault. This was my worst nightmare, and I am responsible for placing you in harm's way."

Lussi took another sip of water. "Don't blame yourself, Sylvia. I disobeyed your instructions. You told me to stop, but I needed answers that could only be found in Oliver Turner's medical records."

"So, you think it was your request for the records that precipitated the attack?"

"I know it was."

"How can you be so sure?"

"Because I know who injected me with fentanyl."

"You saw your attacker?"

"No. She spoke to me, and I recognized her voice."

"Oh, my God. Who was it?"

"My office manager, Barbara Melnick. I can't make sense of it. We work well together, and she's been an invaluable asset to our division."

"Have you told anyone else?"

"No."

"Good. But obviously, this places you in an extremely vulnerable position, Lussi. Presumably, Barbara Melnick was so certain the drug would kill you that she thought there was no risk in revealing her identity."

"She did tell me she'd given me a large dose of fentanyl," Lussi murmured, reaching again for her water glass.

"You were transferred to the PICU directly from the medical records department and I have asked the staff who were involved to keep your admission strictly under wraps. I'm sorry I couldn't allow your family to remain with you. The risk of their being recognized by someone involved in *Broken Hearts* is too high. I need to act quickly to apprehend Ms. Melnick and get you safely out of here. Meanwhile, I have plainclothes officers positioned at strategic points inside and outside the hospital."

"The staff is obeying your instructions, Sylvia. They won't tell me anything and, since Howard and the kids left, you are the only person they have allowed in here. Would you at least tell me how I survived – who resuscitated me?"

"It was Ann Castle, Lussi. She tells me that you even instructed her how to treat you. I've got to leave now, but I'll fill you in on more details when I return."

"If it's any help, Sylvia, Barbara Melnick lives close to the hospital; she walks to work. But I'm sorry, I can't remember her address."

"Obtaining her address should be no problem, Lussi. If she provided valid information when she was hired and remains unaware that you are alive, we have an excellent chance for a speedy arrest. I'll get on with the job now and allow you to rest your voice."

Chapter 23

Thursday, March 26th, 1987, 11:10 a.m.

ANN CASTLE WAS ARRANGING LONG-STEM YELLOW ROSES in a vase on the locker next to Lussi's bed. "I'm relieved to see you looking so much better Lussi. When we left you in the PICU I honestly wondered if you would survive. After that, absolutely no follow-up information was provided to me or the docs on the code blue team, and we were not allowed to return to the PICU in case we inadvertently led the perpetrator there. I was told approximately forty-five minutes ago that you were out of our PICU and had been transferred to Johns Hopkins. I feel privileged to be one of the few who know you are here. I got detailed instructions from the police on how to make certain I wasn't followed."

"I am so glad you are here Ann. I've been told I owe my life to you."

Ann left her flower arranging to take the chair at Lussi's bedside "You saved yourself, Lussi. You told me that you needed Narcan; if you hadn't, I might not have discovered that you had been given an opioid overdose."

"Was anyone with me when you arrived in medical records?"

"No, not a soul. The medical records clerk appeared from a back room after I called the Code Blue. She said she was unaware that anything was going on until she heard the Code announced on the overhead pager."

"Was I breathing when you arrived in medical records?"

"No. At first glance, I thought you'd fallen asleep, but that didn't make sense – you'd just spoken to me on the phone. When I got close enough, I saw that your lips were blue – your pulse was weak and slow. I got you onto the floor and did CPR until the code team arrived. One of the docs intubated your airway while I gave the first dose of Narcan, and the other doc continued the chest compressions. Within a minute of the Narcan injection, you started to take shallow breaths and your color improved a little, but that didn't last long. A few minutes later you stopped breathing again, so we had to give you another dose of Narcan. It took us almost an hour to stabilize you enough to take you to the PICU. You wouldn't believe how many times we had to give you Narcan Lussi. I almost panicked when the first dose wore off so fast – I thought I'd miscalculated the adult dose. You must have received a huge dose of fentanyl. When we moved you to the PICU you were breathing on your own, but you were still unconscious."

Lussi was almost weeping. "I can't tell you how grateful I am to you, Ann."

"Think nothing of it, Lussi – you know you would do the same for me *and* I couldn't have done it without the code team. Has your family visited since you were transferred over here?"

"No. I've spoken by telephone to Howard and the kids. The police have asked them not to visit because they are possibly being watched. They can't even call from home in case the house is bugged."

"That must be very hard for all of you to handle. Do you or do the police have any idea who did this to you Lussi?"

I can't tell you about Barbara – I'm so sorry. "No. Whomever it was must have left almost as you arrived Ann. The only way that I can figure they got away in time to avoid running into you was that they turned right outside the records room and used the hospital exit facing the loading dock. If you use the stairs or the elevator at the left end of the corridor, I don't think there is a direct line of sight down the corridor to that exit door."

"I took the stairs, and you are right, Lucy – I went back today and double-checked. From the foot of the stairs, the corridor deviates to the right, around the entrance to Radiation Oncology. I couldn't even see the entrance to Medical Records. It makes sense too that the perpetrator wouldn't want to be caught inside the hospital with the injection paraphernalia.

"At the time, the police couldn't figure out how the person responsible for assaulting you had escaped without me seeing them. So, they took the medical records clerk away for questioning and she didn't return while I was there."

"You and I need to complete the review of Oliver's records as soon as I get out of here, Ann. If it is worth killing for, information in his file must be key to unraveling *Broken Hearts*."

Ann's face flushed. "When I arrived in medical records, Lussi, there were pages that turned out to have come from Oliver's file, scattered on the desk and floor, but the file itself has disappeared."

Lussi's face fell. "Thank goodness I separated out the nursing notes – all may not be lost."

The end of visiting hours was announced on overhead speakers.

"Lussi, try not to think about *Broken Hearts* until you have recovered from all the trauma you've been through. The police have the pages you took from the file – let them decide if, when, and where it might be safe for us to look at them. I'm off now to find you some distracting reading matter. I'll get one of your nurses to deliver it to you."

Ann stood, reached to retrieve her coat from the back of the chair, and looked intently at Lussi.

Sandwiched between her IV poles, Lussi felt vulnerable and inadequate.

"Ann, have you ever been sure that you've forgotten some vital clue that was right in front of you, but didn't register at the time? Something that could help you make a diagnosis faster or spare a patient an uncomfortable test, for example?"

"Sure, I have Lussi. I think most of us in healthcare regularly use the retro-spectroscope to chastise ourselves but realistically, no matter how hard we strive for it, perfection isn't always achievable."

"In this case, Ann, I don't yet know the outcome. However, I am certain that, if I could just remember what I've forgotten, it would provide crucial information regarding yet-to-be-recognized ringleaders in the *Broken Hearts* conspiracy."

Ann said gently, "Give yourself a break Lussi. If you stop flagellating yourself and relax, you may find the memory returns. If it doesn't, then no foul – you did the best you could. I think you have a rescuer complex, and you are far too courageous for your own good my dear. It must be a Scandinavian thing – you guys are always doing crazy, dangerous stuff like climbing frozen waterfalls and skiing out of airplanes."

Lussi was laughing uncontrollably as Ann replaced her coat and turned to the bedside cabinet.

"I'll just make these flowers more presentable before I leave. Is there anything else I can bring you when I visit next time Lussi? Your favorite candy – fruit? I can't tell you exactly when I'll be back, but I shall nag until I get permission."

"Ouch – I know how effectively you nag Ann. I don't envy the recipient. I'm hoping to be discharged soon, but I would love something non-medical to read."

Chapter 24

Monday, April 6th, 1987, 5.09 p.m.

IT WAS ONE OF THOSE RARE OCCASIONS WHEN LUSSI arrived home from work before other family members. She poured herself a generous glass of wine, kicked off her shoes, stacked pillows against an arm of the couch, and lay down. Having no residual physical injury, she returned to work five days after the fentanyl attack. The official reason provided for her absence was asthmatic bronchitis – a condition she had suffered from periodically since childhood.

Despite the apprehension and arrest of Barbara Melnick just two days after the attack, Lussi found the lack of awareness of whom she should and should not trust at the hospital nerve-wracking. By her third day back at work she had resumed her habit of eating lunch in her office, frequently accompanied by Ann Castle.

Draining her wine glass in less than five minutes, Lussi got up and made for the kitchen to pour a refill.

Whoa, what am I doing? I look forward to relaxing with wine when I get home from work, but I drank that glass so fast I didn't even taste it. I'm relying on wine as an excuse to relax and think, but all can think about is refilling my glass. I need to get out of here.

Gilding the Sherwood Gardens in gold, the late afternoon sun bestowed an unworldly quality. Well-known in Baltimore for the magnificent tulip display in April, Lussi was surprised to find herself almost alone. The six-acre gardens were only three blocks from her home and afforded her a favorite secluded bench, perfect for quiet contemplation.

Removing her coat, Lussi slung it over the back of the bench to cushion her back and proceeded to mentally review recent events and discoveries in *Broken Hearts*.

Barbara confessed to attempted murder soon after her arrest but steadfastly refuses to incriminate anyone else and will not divulge her motive or reveal what has become of Oliver Turner's medical file.

Sylvia Parker is distancing herself from me because, she says, she does not want me placed in danger again. She has indicated that she will make the nursing data removed from Oliver's file available for review – but she hasn't followed through yet.

Thankfully, my notebook was found under the table in medical records, so I have a detailed record of what I discovered prior to the fentanyl injection. Sylvia used my theory on how Oliver's death was fabricated and how he was removed from the hospital to interrogate Azad Sula. His confession matched my theory in almost every detail but, despite Azad's refusal to implicate anyone else, Sylvia is convinced that he was following instructions from higher-ranking conspirators, probably under threat.

Christian Carter's trial is set for May second.

The hunt for the killer of Bill Schultz has stalled. Tony Blake remains the number one suspect, but his wife continues to insist that he was having dinner with her and friends at the time that Bill was shot, and, apparently, the other witnesses continue to back up her story.

Susanne Sinclair, who remains a missing person of interest, has been excluded as a suspect, on the basis that her movements around the time of the murder were witnessed and recorded by police officers. The time gap separating her arrival home and her appearance on the front lawn of the Shultz residence was too brief to allow her to get into position and fire the two shots at Bill Schultz.

Dr. Paul Kader is, apparently, back in Saudi Arabia. His extradition, in exchange for Dr. Azad Sula, was denied last week by the King of Saudi Arabia. There is mounting evidence that Kader was responsible for supplying live donor infants to the heart transplant unit from an unknown source in Saudi Arabia. Kader's 'research' laboratories at South Baltimore Hospital served as a state-of-the-art organ donor/recipient matching facility.

Progress in the case does seem frustratingly slow but, when I review what is known the pieces are starting to fall into place. If only I could recharge my memory.

Lussi glanced at her watch. *I'd better get home; everyone will be home for dinner tonight.*

As Lussi gathered her purse and coat, a woman wearing a silk headscarf and dark glasses appeared from behind the bench, nodded to Lussi, and sat down beside her.

Lussi was surprised – she was rarely disturbed in this out-of-the-way spot and dusk was beginning to fall. She smiled at the intruder and arose to leave.

"Be kind enough to remain here for a little longer, Lussi – I guarantee it will be worth your while."

Lussi immediately recognized the voice.

"Suzanne?"

"Yes."

"Where have you been? The police are searching for you, and I think you can imagine how your husband is feeling."

"Yes indeed. I feel bad about George, but the situation demanded my immediate departure."

"What do you mean by 'the situation'? Did you kill Bill Schultz?"

"No, I most certainly did not. I cannot answer any further questions, Lussi. However, if you can be trusted not to raise an alarm, I have valuable information to share with you which may help the police identify his killer."

"Why are you informing me, Suzanne, rather than the police?

"That has to do with the *situation* that I mentioned, Lussi. Basically, because I trust you to use the information wisely and because I would like to see his killer caught. Do you want to hear what I have for you?"

There is no one close enough to hear me even if I were to scream. Suzanne would hardly have placed herself in such a vulnerable position for no good reason and Sylvia doesn't think she killed Schultz. But she may be armed."

Lussi nodded. "OK. Go ahead."

"It's complicated and you are already aware of some of it, but I shall keep my information as concise as possible. It concerns two individuals involved in the infant heart transplant conspiracy. Paul Kader and Barbara Melnick. I am unable to reveal how I came by this information but hope it will serve to oil the wheels of justice.

"In his childhood, Bill Schultz lived for some time in Saudi Arabia and befriended Paul Kader at school. Kader is one of the many cousins of the Saudi King and has a PhD. in Biochemistry. His first-born son died at the age of five weeks of a complicated heart condition that apparently runs in the male line of the Saudi royal family. Sometime later, Kader's sister-in-law became pregnant with her third child, who turned out to have the same heart condition.

"Kader had apparently learned by this time that Christian Carter was claiming that he could save babies with this heart defect *and* promise them a normal life. He proposed to perform a heart transplant soon after birth, rather, I understand, than first doing a temporizing procedure and then waiting months for the patient to grow before transplanting a new heart. The major obstacle to his approach was the unavailability of infant-size live donor hearts. However, Kader was able to locate a compatible donor for his nephew at an orphanage in Riyadh, and, working through Bill Schultz, both his sister-in-law and the donor infant were covertly transferred to South Baltimore Hospital. These babies were the first to be operated on by Christian Carter at the illicit transplant unit."

I didn't want to believe Alka, but this is exactly what she warned me about. Lussi's horror must have registered on her face because Suzanne stopped speaking and leaned back with a questioning expression on her face.

"So, we have Kader's nephew in our NICU?"

"Yes."

"Why hasn't the family claimed him?"

"I don't know for certain, but I guess it has something to do with the murder charges and the family's reputation. In addition, Kader and Schultz were already involved in a clandestine international operation, set up by the CIA, to launder Saudi money through the United States banking system for the purpose of purchasing weapons for the Mujahideen rebels in Afghanistan to use against the Russia-backed government."

This all fits. "Do you know the location of the orphanage in Riyadh, Suzanne?"

"No. I'm sorry, Lussi, I don't. My time is limited. We need to move on to Barbara Melnick."

"You know she tried to kill me? How do you know?"

Suzanne's voice betrayed some frustration as she replied, "As I told you at the start of this conversation, Lussi, I cannot reveal my sources. Suffice it to say that we need to move on with some alacrity and go our separate ways. So, although Barbara Melnick is not her real name, strangely she chose a false surname that is quite common in Ukraine, her actual country of origin.

"Barbara was born in Southern Ukraine during a man-made famine known as the Holodomor. The Bolsheviks killed millions of Ukrainians by removing their harvested crops and leaving them to starve to death. As a result of surviving the Holodomor, Barbara grew up hating the Russians. She was recruited by the CIA in her twenties. Some contact at Children's Hospital, I do not know their identity, must have notified Barbara about the open position of Office Manager in your division, Lussi. It might have been Bill Shultz, but I have no proof of this. Anyway, her sterling and, surprisingly, valid qualifications ensured that she was hired."

"Yes, she clearly stood out as the best candidate, and she was excellent at her job. Why did she try to kill me?"

"Because, Lussi, somewhere along the line, she'd been inducted into the Saudi/CIA money laundering scheme. You threatened her opportunity for revenge – to do real damage to the Russians by helping the Mujahideen kill their troops in Afghanistan."

So that's what Barbara meant by her *Cause*. I've got a copy of her application material in my office at work, Suzanne. Maybe her list of referees would be helpful?"

"Possibly so."

Darkness had fallen. Suzanne stood abruptly. As she strode away, she called back over her shoulder, "I trust you will not be so foolish as to try to follow me, Lussi. Keep an eye on George for me, but please *do not* tell him I was here."

Chapter 25

Tuesday, April 7th, 1987, 7:16 a.m.

Lussi was back on her bench, this time with Sylvia Parker. She'd met Sylvia at the main gate of the Johns Hopkins University campus, and they'd crossed Charles Street to walk to the Gardens.

"Amazingly, this is the first time I have visited these gardens, Lussi. Although I have wanted to see the famed tulips, something has always gotten in the way. I shall return in a few days when the tulips are in full bloom and, hopefully, it is a bit warmer." Sylvia wrapped her coat around the front of her legs.

Lussi smiled. "This bench is my 'rumination place'. I discovered it shortly after we moved to Guilford – it's a great place to ponder life's problems."

Sylvia laughed. "It sounds like you are about to provide me with plenty to ponder; I may need to borrow it."

Sylvia listened intently while Lussi described her encounter with Suzanne, occasionally scribbling a brief note in a small leather-bound notebook retrieved from her coat pocket. When Lussi had completed her account Sylvia rose from the bench, circled it slowly three times then reclaimed her seat.

"Well, my first question must be how on earth did Suzanne know you were here Lussi? Do you routinely check who's in the near vicinity when you visit this place?

Did you ever mention it to Suzanne?"

"There are rarely many people over in this part of the park, so I've got out of the habit of checking unless I pass several people obviously headed this way. And, I am certain I have never mentioned my bench to Suzanne."

"Did you at any time feel that you were being followed?"

"No. I had no reason to suspect I might be. It was broad daylight in familiar surroundings, and I made the decision to go on impulse. Considering our police guards are no longer considered necessary, I saw no risk."

"Until the killer of Bill Shultz is arrested Lussi, there remains some degree of elevated risk. Granted, we have located, identified, and are dealing with, a good number of the perpetrators involved in *Broken Hearts,* but, as to who might have murdered Schultz, all we have done to date is rule out suspects."

"What about Barbara Melnick? Isn't she a suspect? "

"No, Barbara has a watertight alibi for the time of his murder. And now I've heard Suzanne's information on her, I don't think she has a motive. Bill Schultz was a key player in the Saudi – CIA money laundering scheme – a cash cow for Barbara's revenge on the Russians. Why would she want to slaughter the cow?"

"So why the attempt on my life? Was she working alone? She implied that I was a threat to her cause. How could I be if I wasn't aware that she had one?"

"Key questions Lussi. All I can tell you is that, although Barbara claims that she was working solo, her demeanor when interrogated strongly suggests that she is protecting others. Besides, weren't her words 'our cause', not '*my* cause'?"

"You are correct Sylvia, my error."

"Further to what I was saying, it is of great interest, especially in light of the information provided by Suzanne, that prior to about eleven years ago Barbara Melnick did not exist. She has no passport, driving license, postal address, school record, or bank account that dates back further than nineteen seventy-five. This leads me to wonder if she might be a spy. A sleeper agent placed here to assimilate and adopt the American way of life in readiness to act immediately when ordered to by the foreign entity for whom she is working."

"Isn't it strange that the CIA hasn't answered that question already, Sylvia?"

"Yes, on the face of it. But this case is a quagmire of competing interests. The CIA will only share information when it is in their best interest to do so."

"What about Paul Kader? Knowing now about his royal connections it seems hopeless to think he will ever be tried and punished for his horrifying role in *Broken Hearts*. Now that we know that the first donor infant came from an orphanage in Riyadh, what do you think are the chances of locating it?"

"Well, this should be on the positive side of the CIA coin. With them involved, I think the chances are good. I assume the United States has plenty of their own agents in Saudi Arabia, so take heart Lussi."

"I suppose it would be naive of me to think that the Saudis might exchange Kader for his infant nephew?"

"No, not entirely, Lussi. If his sister-in-law is married to someone higher up in rank in the Saudi Royal Family than Kader that might be possible. However, if the parents request that their son be returned to Saudi Arabia, I don't think that it would do the world image of this country much good to use their baby as a negotiating tool."

"Thank you for agreeing to meet me here Sylvia. I admit that, as time passes, I have tended to let my guard down outside the hospital, but I will be more careful. I have a lecture to give in twenty minutes over at the university, so I had better get going."

"That's fine Lussi and thank *you* for transmitting Suzanne's information. That woman intrigues me. She's a moral chimera – an amoral lifestyle but with signs of a conscience. Of course, what appears to be a conscience could just be self-interest. Anyway, I've put out another BOLO on her, so we shall see."

Chapter 26

Monday, April 20th, 1987, 7:10 a.m.

Spring had cast her revitalizing mantle over the streets of east Baltimore. As Lussi drove to Children's Hospital, she felt relaxed and cheerful, in anticipation of an industrious day setting up her new laboratory at the Children's Hospital Research Institute. As time passed, the detrimental impact of *Broken Hearts* on the morale of the hospital staff had diminished, and things felt almost back to normal, apart from a notable reduction in officious micro-management by those in the executive suite. This welcome change was probably related to the fact that all the current senior management personnel were filling vulnerable interim positions.

Lussi had just one meeting on her morning schedule – following that the workday was hers. Although several key questions relating to *Broken Hearts* remained unanswered, including the identity of Bill Schulz's killer, the orphanage in Riyadh had been located. As it turned out, at least five infants had been abducted from this institution by Paul Kader. However, whether such activity was considered criminal in Saudi Arabia remained indeterminate. Under the protection of the Saudi King, Kader was unlikely to receive appropriate punishment and the identities of the abducted orphans would likely never be revealed.

Kader's nephew was to be returned next week to his parents in Saudi Arabia. On receiving this news, they immediately made a large donation to Children's Hospital for the care of uninsured patients. That donation was to be the topic of the emergency meeting Lussi was attending at eight-thirty a.m. Since learning of the donation, she had been struggling with the morality of accepting what she could only regard as dirty money, versus refusing the donation and depriving sick, underprivileged children of much-needed financial support. She had not reached a palatable conclusion, nor had several other members of the Ethics Committee. The formal meeting of the Ethics committee was scheduled for two days hence. The Committee Chair had pulled together an informal discussion group of undecided committee members and the director of the Chaplaincy service, a Jesuit Priest, had agreed to join them.

9:55 a.m.

AS LUSSI ANTICIPATED, THE MEETING HAD ALREADY RUN into overtime. The Chaplain opened the meeting with an excellent overview of the ethical issues surrounding the donation, and the ensuing discussion was animated, but Lussi feared it would take the judgment of Solomon to achieve consensus. For her, the key to the decision rested on how much the parents of Kader's nephew knew about the source of the donor heart for their son, and she was unlikely to ever know the answer to this question. On the other hand, Lussi did not believe in original sin, so in her view, the heart recipient was as innocent as the donor. The recipient could also be considered a victim, on the basis that he involuntarily underwent an unapproved surgical procedure that had never been performed before on a human infant of his age and size.

Now on her third cup of coffee, Lussi and five of the other eight committee members seated around the table remained undecided.

By the third anonymous vote, two individuals had changed their vote; one from 'undecided' to 'accept the money', the other from 'undecided' to 'don't accept the money'.

Joe Meridian had generously offered his relatively spacious office for the meeting, but was, at this juncture, frequently checking his watch and shifting in his chair.

As the time neared ten fifteen Joe raised his hand. "I apologize guys, but I have another meeting at ten thirty and I must gather up the material I need to take with me. You are welcome to carry on the discussion here in my absence."

There were murmurs of gratitude for the use of the room, as someone suggested a final vote before Joe had to leave. Blank squares of paper were distributed – Joe took his over to his desk, scribbled on it hastily, folded it, and was the first to place it in the bowl at the center of the table. He then proceeded to stuff items from his desk into his briefcase, as the chaplain counted the votes.

Joe closed his briefcase, grabbed his suit jacket from the back of his desk chair, and inserted his right arm into the sleeve. With his back to the desk, he swung to the left to insert his other arm. As the Chaplain was revealing that the results of the fourth vote were identical to the third, the back flap of Joe's jacket snagged a box on his desk. When the box hit the floor, a cascade of small colorful objects escaped and scattered.

Noting the limited remaining time for Joe to get to his next meeting, Lussi said, "Go ahead and leave Joe. We'll pick them up."

As he hurriedly left the room, Joe called, "Thanks guys, great discussion."

The director of pediatric psychiatry bent to retrieve one of the objects from the floor. Grinning like a schoolboy he exclaimed, "These are really great pencil-top erasers, much nicer than the ones we buy for the kids in our clinic."

He strode over and picked up the box from the floor, scrutinized the outside, and replaced it on the desk, before tearing a sticky note off a pad and recording information from the box lid.

Kneeling, Lussi picked up a handful of erasers. There were at least ten different animals, all less than two inches tall. Each had an opening in the base to allow the insertion of the blunt end of a pencil. Sitting back on her heels, Lussi transferred one of the erasers into her pocket and then stood to replace the others in the box, first stirring the contents until she encountered and extracted the specific animal she was searching for. Before following the others out of the room, Lussi also recorded the manufacturer's information.

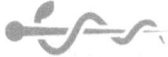

11:08 a.m.

Lussi was waiting for Ann outside the classroom where she was concluding a teaching session.

"Hi Lussi, were you looking for me? I thought you were in the lab today."

"I was supposed to be there, Ann, but something has come up. Do you have time to talk?"

"Well, yes, I was just going to take a coffee break, would you like to join me?"

"Do you mind if we take our coffee to my office? I don't want to be overheard."

"Sure, let's do it Lussi."

When she was in her office Lussi rarely locked the door, but this time she did so as soon as Ann and she were inside. Ann looked at her quizzically as she took a seat.

"What's going on Lussi?"

"I'm not one hundred percent certain, Ann, but I think I may be in possession of a significant clue to who killed Bill Shultz."

"Have you remembered what it was you were trying to recall?"

"Yes, Ann, I did finally remember, soon after I stumbled by accident on this additional clue. Just to put you in the picture, Sylvia Parker told me, some time ago, that she was frustrated because the only possibly contemporary item discovered at the site from which the police believe his killer shot Bill Shultz was what she described as a 'child's toy' – a small rubber lion. Well, I have come across a box of similar animal figures that turn out to be erasers that kids put on the ends of their pencils. Now, I need to find out if these are regularly used by any, or all, of the cardiology medical staff. I was wondering if you knew any of the nurses in cardiology well enough to ask them whether all the attending medical staff have and distribute these erasers to the patients, or is this practice confined to a single individual?"

"Have you a suspect in mind Lussi."

"I do, Ann, but it's a long – shot and I don't think it is a good idea to color your perspective in advance. "

Lucy pulled open a desk drawer and extracted a plastic sandwich bag containing the two erasers.

"When you do this, Ann, make sure that you are not overheard by any of the cardiology attendings."

"Of course, I'll do that, Lussi. I know most of the nurses in cardiology. I'll simply say that I like the way these little guys are made and would like to purchase some myself."

"Thank you, Ann. You will need to include nurses that work in the cardiology clinic, as well as those on the inpatient service. I have learned that pencil topper erasers are routinely given to their clinic patients by the psychiatrists, but theirs are not purchased from the same manufacturer."

Chapter 27

Friday, April 24th, 1987, 9:00 a.m.

ONCE AGAIN LUSSI WAS SITTING WITH ANN CASTLE, Sylvia Parker, and Lieutenant Strand around the table in Sylvia's office.

Sylvia reintroduced Lieutenant Strand and then said, "Lieutenant, as I recently informed you, Dr. Sim and Ms. Castle have additional information to share with us regarding the murder of Bill Shultz. I will, therefore, immediately hand over the meeting to them."

"Thanks, Colonel," said Lussi, "the new information that Ann and I have uncovered relates to the pencil eraser animal that was found in the woods behind Bill Shultz's house. I had almost forgotten about this find until, quite by accident, I happened on a box of similar erasers in the office of a colleague."

Sylvia's eyebrows rose. "I sincerely hope you were not ignoring my instructions to quit snooping, Dr. Sim. If you took these erasers from someone's office that you had entered without invitation, that someone could simply deny that the erasers were ever there, and it would be your word against theirs."

"Definitely not, Colonel. I was attending a meeting in the office in question, with nine colleagues. All of us saw the box of erasers fall to the floor when the 'someone' himself accidentally knocked it off his desk."

The Colonel smiled. "I gather you are going to keep the Lieutenant and I in suspense to the bitter end, Dr. Sim."

"Well, Colonel, Ann and I thought it would be best to explain our reasoning before we reveal the suspect. For all we knew at that point, a significant percentage of the hospital staff might own these animal erasers. As it was, the director of psychiatry admitted on the spot that he did."

"OK, that makes sense. I will stop interrupting."

"At this point, I'm going to hand over to Ann to explain how she determined that the eraser was not just a red herring but was a potentially solid piece of evidence – Ann."

"OK. To make a long story short, this week I spoke individually and at different times and locations to several members of the nursing staff on the inpatient and outpatient cardiology service. I showed them two erasers from the suspects' desk and expressed an interest in purchasing similar items. I asked each nurse if they knew of any cardiology staff who routinely distributed them to patients so that I might find out where the erasers could be purchased. In total, I spoke to seven nurses. I must admit, I feared that the erasers would be so commonplace that they would prove useless as evidence, but I was wrong. Three nurses told me they had not noticed anyone distributing them, the other four spontaneously identified the same individual, including one of them who added that this individual 'always had some in his pocket'. I am personally sad to report that the individual they identified was Dr. Joe Meridian."

"Thank you both for your valuable information which, I am relieved to note, you appear to have obtained without putting yourselves at risk. This was a well-planned undertaking with results that we will pursue, but I'm unclear why you restricted your inquiry to the cardiology service. It would seem to me that, before concluding that Dr. Meridian is a suspect, we will first have to expand your inquiry to the remainder of the hospital, Ann. We must rule out others who may distribute these specific erasers. Your conclusion makes sense based on the fact that Dr. Meridian was a consultant involved in the care of Oliver Turner and, albeit briefly, a consultant to the NICU at South Baltimore Hospital. However, we have uncovered no evidence that he was aware of the existence of the transplant unit prior to the raid. Christian Carter has stated on several occasions that Meridian was not involved, and he has not been identified as a co-conspirator by any of the other suspects. So, what might be his motive for killing Shultz?"

"I have information to add, Colonel, which might explain why Ann and I are more confident than it seems we should be that Joe Meridian is a viable suspect in the murder of Bill Schultz. May I explain?"

"Of course, doctor, please do."

"First, I owe you all an apology. I was provided with a clue to Joe's involvement in *Broken Hearts* soon after I returned to work following the sugar factory incident. I am embarrassed to say that I somehow suppressed this evidence, to the point that I could recall that I had encountered vital information, but could not remember what it was, when it was, or how or by whom it was presented. Like Ann, I have considered Joe a true friend and a trustworthy colleague – so maybe I suppressed this information for that reason.

"Anyway, on my first day back at work I now clearly recall Joe asking me if I was suffering any, as he put it, 'residual problems', and at the same time he placed his hand on the back of my head. In retrospect, he was obviously and specifically enquiring about the head injury I sustained in the transplant unit, but I responded as if he had simply asked about my general health. I believe there was no way that he could have known that I was struck on the head during my kidnapping unless he was involved. I recalled this incident only after finding the lion eraser in Joe's office. I fully recognize that if I had told you about this at the time, Colonel, Bill Schultz might still be alive."

There was absolute silence in the room, finally broken by Lieutenant Strand who got to his feet and clapped his hands. Then he addressed Lussi and Ann.

"With apologies to you, Colonel, for breaking protocol, I have to say that since I joined the police force, I have rarely had the good fortune to encounter witnesses of the caliber of Dr. Sim and Nurse Castle. Their integrity, intelligence, work ethic, and perseverance have been demonstrated on multiple occasions over the course of this case, as has their dedication to the well-being of their patients.

"I would like to express my personal gratitude to both of you for the assistance you have provided and state that I feel strongly that neither of you have any reason to feel anything but pride for what you have achieved in this case."

The Lieutenant took his seat. The Colonel's face was inscrutable.

"Well, I'll be darned if that isn't the longest speech, I've ever heard from you, Lieutenant." Said the Colonel, breaking into a broad smile. "I can't say I disagree with you either – another exceptional experience. Joking apart, ladies, I couldn't have said it better myself. I think you may have just handed us the final piece in the *Broken Hearts* jigsaw."

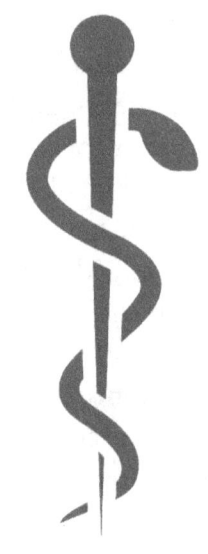

Epilogue

Thursday, November 26th, 1987, 5.15 p.m.

The snowfall had slackened, allowing Lussi to fully appreciate the captivating view of Baltimore Harbor eleven floors below. The rippled, ruby-red reflection of the Domino Sugar sign reached out to her across the harbor, punctuated by scattered white lights on boats at anchor bobbing on the velvet black water. Ringing the scene to the west was an uneven honeycomb of light from the windows of shops, restaurants, and hotels and, close to a docked navy frigate, illuminations on a stationary carousel added a hint of enchantment.

The Sim family and George Sinclair had developed a close friendship in the past six months. They, along with several other guests, were about to enjoy Thanksgiving dinner served in the elegant dining room of his penthouse condominium. There were multiple contributors to the celebration, some of whom had not seen each other for at least six months. For the main course, Donna Shultz prepared the turkey and dressing, and Lussi and Rachel the sauces, sweet potatoes, and greens. For dessert, Sylvia Parker made pumpkin pies and Ann Castle concocted a trifle with multi-colored layers.

Other key duties were assigned to George, Howard, John, and Sylvia's husband, Marcus, who had retired to the pool room when the cooking began. They reappeared a couple of hours later to prepare snacks and drinks for the cooks.

Lussi's reverie at the window was interrupted by the sound of a dinner gong, followed by George requesting that his guests proceed to the dining room.

A wood fire was blazing in the hearth and, beneath the most stunning chandelier Lussi had ever seen, was a table set for royalty.

The food was tasty and the conversation lively but, as the evening progressed, Lussi gained the impression that the guests were intentionally avoiding discussion of the events that had originally brought them together. There were so many moving parts to the *Broken Hearts* conspiracy, requiring complex legal and diplomatic maneuvering, Lussi felt she could not be the only person at the table who still had unanswered questions.

As after dinner drinks were served Lussi seized an opportunity.

"I don't know how you guys feel about this, and I don't want to cast shadows on a happy occasion but do any of you have questions about *Broken Hearts* that you would like answered? All of us were involved in different ways, so I thought maybe we could help each other out by filling in information gaps."

The other guests looked around the table and fidgeted in their chairs, until George, who was standing at a sideboard pouring drinks, spoke up.

"I think that's an excellent idea, Lussi. What about the rest of you? Does anyone object?"

"Then, hearing no objections let's go ahead. Lussi, would you like to start us off?"

"Thank you, George. As most of you know, I was completely taken in by Joe Meridian. His leadership role in *Broken Hearts* was a massive, unforgivable betrayal of his patients, their families, his colleagues, and medical ethics. So, after his arrest, I did not want to think about him but, with time, I have become curious about the life path that led an undeniably excellent physician to become involved in an appalling scheme like *Broken Hearts*."

Sylvia took a sip of her brandy. "I'll attempt to answer your question, Lussi. Did I ever tell you that it was Joe who tailgated you to the hospital on the night that Oliver Turner was admitted to Children's Hospital? He confessed that he borrowed the limo from his brother-in-law, expressly for the purpose. Apparently, after Dr. Sally Wright broke off the telephone call with you, Ann, she called Joe. Joe told her that he would take care of the situation and would go into Children's to examine Oliver in her stead. Joe obviously didn't know exactly when you would leave home, Lussi, but he knew your car well and was aware of the route you take from home to the hospital. He was waiting for you at an intersection that he knew you would have to pass through on the way."

"I'm not surprised to hear that, Sylvia. I don't suppose he told you why he did it?"

"Not directly, Lussi, but I'm certain Joe meant to scare you so that you would continue to value his support. According to him, he got the idea because you apparently told him, a few days earlier, how upset you were about the gang shooting that killed the mother of the twin boys."

"Yes, Sylvia, I'm afraid I did."

"Well stop feeling bad; this will be interesting to all of you who were deceived by Dr. Meridian. Regarding the role of Dr. Wright in *Broken Hearts,* it turns out she was also an innocent victim. It seems that, far from the charming and dedicated image that Joe Meridian presented to the hospital in general, he was a petty tyrant in his own division. His colleagues lived in fear of falling out of favor. Apparently, Dr. Wright had no idea what was going on at South Baltimore Hospital but did not dare to question Joe's instructions. Punishments received by those more courageous have included not only losing their job but also having their career severely damaged by the negative information widely distributed by Joe."

Lussi was highly animated. "That is fascinating, Sylvia. I have wondered since I started to work at Children's Hospital why the average age of Joe's colleagues was so much lower than in my own or other divisions. People seemed to leave his program as soon as they reached their late thirties. I assumed they moved elsewhere for family reasons, but it was strange that none of his colleagues were promoted to higher positions within his division. Also, it is standard, but not required, that a division director appoint a deputy. As far as I'm aware, Joe never had a second-in-command."

"There you have it Lussi – an explanation for your intuitive hunch," said Sylvia, giving Lussi a thumbs up. "But, to get back to your original question, you know that both Bill Schultz and Joe Meridian were affiliated with the CIA, but in the press and during the trials the CIA have maintained they were contractors, not agents, implying they had more choice regarding the methods they used than do agents, who are CIA employees. This may indeed have been the case by the time they devised the *Broken Hearts* scheme.

Anyway, it seems that the CIA would like the public and the juries to believe that Bill and Joe were working either entirely on their own or, at most, as rogue agents.

"Bill and Joe were recruited by the CIA from wealthy families, with quite different backgrounds, and for quite different reasons. Bill, based on his financial expertise and high-ranking contacts in the Middle East; Joe, based upon his Cuban heritage and his father's long-term service in the CIA. Seemingly, the one thing the two had in common was their hatred for the communists.

"Knowledge of Joe's background has shed light on the link between Lussi's abduction from the transplant unit and the selection of the Domino Sugar factory as the disposal site for her body. Joe was the only child of a sugar magnate in Cuba, prior to the takeover of the government by Fidel Castro in nineteen fifty-nine. Castro, having denied at first that he was a communist, developed close relationships with other communist regimes, including making a sugar pact with Russia.

"One of Castro's first major moves was to confiscate the wealth of those who had supported his ousted predecessor, Fulgencio Batista. This included the nationalization of their sugar plantations and other business property and exile from Cuba. Like the majority of those exiled by Castro, Joe's father went to the United States, where he was recruited, along with other high-level Cuban exiles, by the CIA. These recruits provided clandestine information on Castro and the 'Cuba Problem.'

"It seems that Joe's father never fully regained the wealth and position he had enjoyed in Cuba, but he was employed in senior management positions in the United States sugar refining industry. As a teen, Joe spent a considerable portion of his summer vacations working in sugar processing plants, including the Domino plant here in Baltimore. At that time, he apparently talked openly about his hatred of Castro and the communists for robbing him of the splendid future in Cuba that he should be inheriting from his father."

Lussi commented, "So, Joe was familiar with the layout of the Domino Sugar hangar. The same hangar has been there for decades. This explains how the people who captured me knew where to place me on the conveyor belt, but apparently not the details of the working time schedule for the belt. I am sure they did not anticipate that the belt would shut down before I was under a mound of sugar."

"Yes, exactly, Lussi. We know that the CIA recruited Joe at the age of twenty-seven when he was finishing his medical school training, but at that point the CIA information trail is blocked. We know that his CIA assignment at Children's Hospital was to keep an eye on Bill Schultz, but nothing about his prior assignments."

"But why did Joe need to keep an eye on Bill?" Asked Donna. "Didn't the CIA know exactly what Bill was doing? Didn't they get him into the money laundering business in the first place?"

"Yes, Donna, when he became division director of pediatric cardiology at Children's Hospital, Joe was fully aware of Bill's expertise in international money laundering. The CIA briefed him on their suspicions that, rather than assisting the war on communism, Bill was now feathering his own nest. Joe was assigned to uncover the extent of Bill's extracurricular international financial activity. Have I answered your question, Donna?"

"You certainly have, thank you, Sylvia. I can't believe that I was living with Bill while all of this was going on and

I had no idea. I thought I was only dealing with a broken marriage. No wonder he always kept his office locked. He wouldn't even let the cleaning lady in there."

George offered to refill their drinks, before asking the next question.

"Why build the transplant unit? As a businessman, I can think of many less complicated methods to launder money."

"I'll answer that one," said Lussi. "Please, all of you, feel free to interrupt me if I get carried away with the medical stuff.

"Well, it seems that Joe easily gained Bill's trust. He discovered that Bill was working on a deal with the Saudi royal family involving the development of a pediatric heart transplant unit at South Baltimore Community Hospital. Unlike previous deals with the Saudis, this one was not based on the potential for money laundering alone. Apparently, male children born into certain branches of the Saudi royal family have a high incidence of a severe heart defect known as hypoplastic left heart syndrome, which is present from birth.

"The deal was, that if Bill and Christian Carter supervised the design and construction of the transplant facility, using Saudi money, Dr. Kader guaranteed that compatible live donor infants would be provided for Carter's future transplant patients from orphanages in Saudi Arabia.

"Recognizing the potential financial benefits, Joe was eager to participate as a full partner and, naturally, neglected to inform his CIA handlers about his plans.

I had come to believe it was Joe who hit me on the head in the transplant unit, but it turns out it was Paul Kader."

The listeners exchanged glances in silence.

Ann asked, "Why did they need Oliver Turner, Lussi if they had a supply of heart donors?"

"Well, as you know, Ann, the first infant on Christian Carter's surgical list was Paul Kader's nephew. Am I correct in saying that the donor of his heart has been traced, Sylvia?"

Sylvia nodded. "Yes. The CIA was able to locate the orphanage in Riyadh where Paul Kader found a heart donor for his son. Even though his son died before this donor could be used, there was information on his origin in Kader's son's medical records, and the CIA was able to confirm that the donor infant for Kader's nephew came from the same orphanage. Sadly, the parents of this infant cannot be located, and we believe that his body was eventually disposed of in the incinerator at South Baltimore Hospital."

"Thanks, Sylvia. To get back to Ann's question, we know that one of the four infants rescued from the transplant unit was the originally intended donor for the second heart transplant, which was scheduled for the day of the raid. This infant is of Arabic ethnicity, but efforts to track down his parents have met bureaucratic roadblocks. Azad Sula testified that this donor was sent to the United States having been tissue typed in Saudi Arabia. However, on repeat tissue typing at Kader's lab, he didn't prove a perfect match with the baby requiring a heart, who was not doing well. So, a new donor had to be found quickly and Kader began to tissue type every baby born at South Baltimore Hospital. Eventually, he found a perfect match in Oliver Turner."

George stood up and stretched. "My sincere apologies. This discussion is both horrifying and fascinating, and I'm hesitant to interrupt, but my back is insisting I find another seat. Shall we take a break and move to the living room where the chairs are more comfortable?"

Donna led the way to the living room.

John asked the next question. "I know Dr. Meridian and Dr. Sula made baby Turner sick and then sneaked him out of Children's Hospital. How did they do it without anyone suspecting anything?"

"As you know, John, attempting to answer this question got your mother into serious trouble, so I think that she is the person to provide your answer," Sylvia observed. "Because Joe Meridian has proved such an uncooperative witness, he has slowed the process of confirming what your mother figured out months ago. Lussi, are you willing to go ahead?"

"That's fine, but it is a complicated story. Please feel free to ask questions along the way.

"On the morning that Oliver's condition suddenly deteriorated, Dr. Azad Sula examined him with the cardiologists in the ECMO room. After they had completed this examination, Azad ran through a series of alternative settings on Oliver's ventilator. He then returned the ventilator to the original settings, so that there was no need to order the respiratory therapist to make a permanent change. Under cover of fiddling with the ventilator settings, and with prior direction from Joe Meridian, Azad surreptitiously detached the tube feeding oxygen into the back of Oliver's ventilator, before leaving the room to make rounds in the NICU. So that Oliver's nurse would not look at the oxygen flow meter on the wall and realize that the flow rate to her patient was zero, Azad left the oxygen flowing into the room through the detached tubing.

"Joe calculated that, because Oliver was still receiving oxygenated blood from the ECMO pump, albeit at minimal flow, his deterioration in clinical status would be slowed. Joe figured this would give him time to intervene after Azad left the ECMO room and to reattach the oxygen tube to the ventilator when it became necessary to save Oliver's life.

"The circulation of our blood when we are a fetus in the womb is a little different from the circulation after we are born. This is because, in the womb, the placenta does the work of the lungs, so that blood does not need to flow through the fetal lungs to provide oxygen and remove carbon dioxide. A small blood vessel called the *ductus arteriosus* allows blood to bypass the lungs while we are a fetus but must close after birth to allow blood to flow through our lungs.

"In the first few days of life, a significant drop in the blood oxygen will frequently cause the *ductus arteriosus* to reopen, causing heart failure and a drop in blood pressure. This is what happened to Oliver when his oxygen supply through the ventilator was interrupted by Azad Sula.

"When Joe entered the ECMO room to consult on the two patients that morning, he brought with him a vial of prostaglandin. He did this for two reasons. First, because he knew that as soon as he reattached the oxygen tubing to the back of his ventilator Oliver would probably recover quickly because his ductus would close in response to correcting the level of oxygen in his blood. This did not fit his plan. Joe needed Oliver to remain compromised, but not to the point where he could not be resuscitated, or the lack of oxygen might cause damage to his heart. The second indication for the prostaglandin was to keep his ductus open long enough to obtain X-ray and ultrasound verification of Joe's diagnosis.

"So, Joe instructed his cardiology team to leave the ECMO room and complete rounds in the NICU without him. As soon as they left, he administered the prostaglandin intravenously to keep Oliver's ductus open, having previously led both his medical team and Oliver's nurse to believe that he was intending to administer indomethacin to close his ductus.

"Unfortunately for Joe. Oliver's nurse was too smart for him. Correct me if I am wrong Sylvia, but I understand she testified she saw Joe administering the prostaglandin and asked what it was. Joe indicated by a gesture that he could not hear her and was too involved in the resuscitation to pause. I guess he thought she would forget about it with all that was going on. The ECMO pump technician, trying to be helpful, did respond to the nurse, telling her that it was *probably* indomethacin. However, Oliver's nurse later retrieved the vial, which she saw Joe dispose of in the receptacle for used needles, and she documented the dose of prostaglandin in the nursing record. Joe never thought, it appears, that anyone would be sufficiently conscientious to go hunting for the vial in a disposal box full of contaminated needles."

Ann Castle allowed her pent-up anger to explode. "Joe should have known better than to underestimate our nurses. How could he think that Oliver's nurse would overlook the precise identification of a drug given to her patient? I keep asking myself how on earth I didn't recognize long ago what an amoral jerk he is."

"Everyone was taken in by him, Ann, especially me." Said Lussi. "This information is upsetting and it's getting late. Do you guys want me to continue? We could finish this some other time?"

To Lussi's surprise, there was enthusiastic consensus that she should continue.

"OK. I know that what I'm telling you must be hard for those without training in healthcare to follow. Please don't hesitate to ask questions.

"Recovery from the malignant treatment Oliver had received from Azad and Joe would be slow. Joe and Azad continued the charade that they were attempting to resuscitate him so that, although not actually dead, as he was finally pronounced by Joe, when Oliver's parents arrived Oliver's skin would be pale and swollen and he would not appear to them to be alive. It was not included in the medical or nursing record, but Oliver's nurse testified in court that sometime before Joe stopped the resuscitation, Azad tripped on an electrical cord and fell against the stand holding the heart and respiration monitor. The monitor crashed to the floor. Azad quickly examined the monitor, declared that it was no longer functional, and left it unplugged. Thus, there was, from that time onward, no evidence to an observer that Oliver had a heartbeat, and his body was so swollen that even the breaths he was receiving from the ventilator produced almost undetectable movement of his chest. According to Oliver's nurse, Joe immediately 'came to the rescue' by, quote, 'using the most reliable monitor', and proceeding to replace the heart monitor with his stethoscope until he terminated the resuscitation a short time later."

George was visibly shocked. "The poor little guy; how did they get him out of there without someone noticing he was still breathing?"

"Joe had the whole exit process carefully planned. Azad rushed the grieving parents in and out of the ECMO room as quickly as possible, only allowing them to briefly touch Oliver after providing them with misinformation about his lines and tubes. Joe had previously distributed copies of a research protocol titled, *Outcome of male versus female infants on ECMO* and informed the nursing staff erroneously that Oliver's parents had agreed to allow him to enter this study. The protocol required that only the senior researchers, which included Azad and himself, could record research data while they *personally,* rather than the nursing staff, removed the deceased patient from ECMO and prepared the body for transfer to Pathology. In fact, this research project had never been ratified by the Institutional Research Committee, but with the nursing staff out of the room, Joe and Azad could remove Oliver from ECMO after clamping his ECMO cannulas, provide him with oxygen from a mobile oxygen tank, and hand ventilate him with a bag until he was out of the building.

"Waiting outside Children's Hospital was an ambulance containing staff from South Baltimore Hospital, who placed Oliver on a ventilator and provided intensive care, including indomethacin to close his ductus, on the way to the transplant unit.

"We now know that the body taken to Pathology by Dr. Azad was that of the infant who donated his heart to Paul Kader's nephew. Azad transferred Oliver's identification bracelet to his body. He had earlier inserted ECMO cannulas into his neck and clamped them. There was an unhealed incision on the donor's chest relating to the removal of his heart. However, the staff member receiving the body in Pathology would not be aware of the details of Oliver's surgical history or able to recognize, from external examination, that the heart was missing.

"Joe, with the help of my office manager, Barbara Melnick, made sure that the patient switch would never be discovered by arranging for someone claiming to be the undertaker to pick up the body of the donor infant soon after arrival in Pathology. The admission and discharge paperwork was completed, and the body was transferred to the phony undertaker before the assigned freezer space was ever used. Are there any questions?"

"Mom, why did Barbara help Joe?" John asked. "The times I met her in your office, she was always so nice to me. It is hard to imagine her being mixed up in this."

"Apparently John, Barbara met Joe when they were both in Russia working undercover for different countries. When they were children, both of their families suffered hardship related to the Russian communists – as a result, both hated the Russians. Barbara was fully aware of the role of the CIA in the laundering of money to arm the Mujahedeen rebels to fight the Russians in Afghanistan and wanted to ensure that the flow of money continued. Joe helped her to get hired as my office manager and, from that time on, she did everything that Joe asked her to, including the attack on me with fentanyl. Does that make things clearer?"

"Yes, it does, thanks, Mom."

When no one else indicated they had questions, Lussi stood and walked over to George. She whispered something in his ear, and they left the room together.

Donna Shultz was cradling a cup of coffee. "I've never heard the whole story of how and why Joe killed my husband. I guess I wanted to avoid dredging up unpleasant memories, so I've never asked for details. But now I've heard all this background information I find myself wanting to hear more."

"I'm happy to tell you all we know, Donna." Said Sylvia. "Joe Meridian is one of our least cooperative perpetrators, to say the least. Now that his true personality is revealed it is clear how selfish, entitled, and resentful he is. When he's asked a question that he prefers not to answer he responds like a juvenile, sulking and having temper tantrums. But we have persevered and, I think, obtained most of the truth.

"Joe was fully aware that Bill would sell-out his fellow conspirators without hesitation if it served his own best interests. On the day of the shooting, Joe brought his weapon and ammunition to work with him and left them in his car. He had a full day of clinical duties scheduled, which he could not delegate without drawing unwanted attention to himself. He left Children's Hospital in the late afternoon, then drove to your home, Donna. Stopping at a high point on the road, about a quarter of a mile from the rear of your property, he studied your house through binoculars.

"As you are aware, Joe had previously attended several meetings at your home, Donna, and was quite familiar with the inside layout of the first floor, including the location of Bill's office window at the back of the house. Joe told us in his confession that he'd initially planned to shoot Bill at his desk, through this window, but it became clear by the time he was hiding in the trees behind the house that Bill was preparing to leave. His car was parked in your circular driveway, facing the backyard with an open trunk.

"Because he approached your house through the woods at the rear, Joe was not aware that the police were changing shifts at the end of the access road to your and the Sinclair's homes. He stated that, although dusk had fallen by the time he was in place, because of your excellent exterior lighting he had a clear view through his rifle scope past the side of the house to the front driveway.

"Joe saw Bill, with a suitcase in one hand and a coat slung over his other arm, go to the back of his car, put the suitcase in the trunk, and close it. He was prepared to fire as soon as Bill turned to face him and started walking toward the front of his car. However, after taking one or two steps, Bill pulled open the left rear passenger door and leaned into the car to deposit his coat on the back seat. Thus, the first bullet missed the target and Bill ran back to the house.

"Joe further stated that he was preparing to leave, thinking that Bill's wife or a neighbor would call the police. To his surprise, Bill ran back to his car and, while opening the driver's seat door, for some unknown reason turned to face him and froze, offering him a perfect target. The lion pencil eraser could have fallen from Joe's pocket at any time, perhaps while he was retrieving the bullet casings."

The room was silent until John said, 'Wow', and then it seemed to Lussi that everyone exhaled at the same time. She and George had returned to the room after a brief absence. They were standing together near the door when George said, "Lussi tells me she thinks that no one is asking about Suzanne to spare my feelings. I thank you all for showing me so much consideration. Most of you know how much I love my wife. I wish I knew where she is, but every day that I do not learn that she has come to harm I am happy. It will remain that way until we find each other again. I thank you all for the treasured friendship you are sharing with me."

This time the silence lasted longer. Then Donna said, "No one deserves a happy ending more than you do George." At which point he received a standing ovation.

As the clapping receded, Lussi retook her seat. "It's getting late, still snowing, and the roads out there are probably not so good. George tells me he has received multiple offers of help with the washing up and wants me to relieve your consciences by assuring you that he has taken care of it. Paid professionals are accomplishing the task as I speak.

"I don't want to delay anyone's departure for home in this weather, but may I briefly share something which would not have occurred without the support of all of you here?

"When I came to this country, I carried with me unwanted mental baggage. From early childhood, when I felt inadequate to deal with a stressful or threatening situation I reverted, like all of us human animals, to an instinctive survival decision; run away or fight? Over time, the choice vanished, and I was automatically triggered to fight. This continued as an adult, frequently accompanied by flashbacks to and dreams of unpleasant events.

"As you can all probably imagine, this trigger to fight frequently overcame my diplomatic skills. For example, it surfaced during financial discussions with those members of the upper management at Children's Hospital who pressured me to accept funding cuts that I could predict would lead to sub-optimal patient care.

"To cut a long story short, I developed a reputation for being confrontational and constantly felt I was letting down my patients because I lacked the skills necessary to successfully negotiate on their behalf. This, I believe, contributed to my descent under the thrall of Joe Meridian's magnetic personality, and to what I can now clearly recognize was my dependence on him as an emotional crutch. I am not telling you this to garner sympathy – quite the reverse. Because, of course, there are positive uses for anger, and my unwanted baggage proved instrumental in equipping me to survive *Broken Hearts*. I am delighted to report that over the past six months, I have, with expert help, discarded my encumbrance of superfluous guilt and anger and my flashbacks and nightmares have ceased to exist."

www.ingramcontent.com/pod-product-compliance
Lightning Source LLC
LaVergne TN
LVHW041919070526
838199LV00051BA/2669

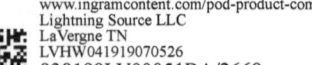